Planning Patient Care

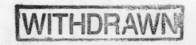

The Editors

Lynn Batehup, BSc, MSc, RGN, is currently Clinical Lecturer in the Department of Nursing Studies, King's College, University of London, and at St George's Hospital.

Jenifer Wilson-Barnett, FRCN, PhD, RGN, is Professor of Nursing Studies at King's College, University of London.

The Contributors

Alison Jesson, RGN, HVCert, is currently Senior Nurse, Cardiac Counsellor and Specialist in Cardiac Rehabilitation at St George's Hospital, London.

Val Thomson, RGN, ADM, PGCEA, MTD, is currently a Midwife Tutor at the London Hospital.

Sue Adams, BSc, RGN, is currently a Sister in the Accident and Emergency Department at St George's Hospital, London.

Gary Tubman, RMN, is currently a Charge Nurse in the Community Psychiatric Department of St George's Hospital, London.

Sally Glen, RGN, RSCN, DN(Lond), RNT, DipEd(Lond), has been awarded a Health Education Council Scholarship and is currently studying at the Institute of Education, London.

Alison While, BSc, MSc, PhD, SRN, HVCert, is currently a Lecturer in the Department of Nursing Studies at King's College, University of London.

The illustrations on the front cover and on pages 1, 19, 45, 53, 67, 79 and 97 are by Duncan Smith.

Planning Patient Care

Edited by

Lynn Batehup

Clinical Lecturer, Department of Nursing Studies
King's College, University of London
and
St George's Hospital, London

and

Jenifer Wilson-Barnett

Professor of Nursing Studies
King's College, University of London

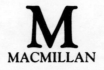

MACMILLAN

First published 1988

Published by
MACMILLAN EDUCATION LTD
Houndmills, Basingstoke, Hampshire RG21 2XS
and London
Companies and representatives
throughout the world

Printed in Hong Kong

ISBN 0–333–46097–9

Contents

The Editors and the Contributors   ii

Introduction   *Lynn Batehup*   vii

1   Rehabilitation after a myocardial infarction: Health education and counselling for long-term recovery   *Alison Jesson*   1

2   Helping a patient to understand diabetes: Teaching plan to promote an independent lifestyle   *Lynn Batehup*   9

3   Assisting a mother to establish breastfeeding: Planning for a happy and successful postnatal period   *Val Thomson*   19

4   A patient who has had cardiac surgery to relieve unstable angina: Planning in the acute recovery stage   *Lynn Batehup*   27

5   An elderly lady who keeps falling: Planning for safe mobility   *Lynn Batehup*   35

6   Symptom control for a patient with breast cancer: Planning for comfort   *Lynn Batehup*   45

7   Drug overdose: Planning sensitive care in the accident and emergency department *Sue Adams and Gary Tubman*   53

8   Recovery from a stroke: Rehabilitation in the acute recovery stage   *Lynn Batehup*   67

9   A patient who has had a lobectomy: Planning in the acute post-operative period *Sally Glen*   79

10   A patient with heart failure: Planning care for a successful recovery   *Jenifer Wilson-Barnett*   87

11   A handicapped child admitted to hospital to improve her mobility skills: Planning care to improve walking and other self-care activities   *Alison While*   97

12   Conclusion   *Lynn Batehup and Jenifer Wilson-Barnett*   105

Index   109

Lynn Batehup

Introduction

Planning patient care involves nurses in systematically assessing for and identifying a patient's problems, setting goals and outcomes, establishing interventions and evaluating the results. Planning is a universal concept that is used to ensure that future actions and results are those that are intended. The care plan is the tool used to document the process, to facilitate communication between care givers and to ensure continuity of care. The format that the care plan takes should be dictated by the needs of the individuals and the setting in which it is to be used. A certain rigidity exists regarding what data should be included in the care plan. There is no format that is more acceptable than any other. The main reason for the inclusion of any type of data in the care plan is that it should facilitate achievement of the patient's goals.

The format that is used for the plans in this book, is based on that proposed by Mayers (1983) and includes:

1. *Assessment* (gathering data, analysis and interpretation).
2. *Identifying problems.*
3. *Defining expected outcomes* (ongoing evaluation criteria).
4. *Prescribing interventions* (after considering options, constraints and resources).
5. *Evaluation* at periodic end point intervals.

Assessment

Planned nursing care begins with an assessment. A thorough assessment provides data to enable the nurse to identify the problem areas. According to Christensen (1982), tools for data collection include interaction, observation and measurement. Making observations rather than drawing conclusions when collecting the data is important. Observations should be objective descriptions of behaviour; a conclusion is an interpretation, and it may therefore not be objective. Conclusions should not be drawn until all the available information is collected. Therefore, when carrying out an assessment, the nurse makes observations and uses communication to obtain information. More objectivity can be achieved if measurement is included, for example tracing and measuring an ulcer, or assessing pain with a pain ruler (Bourbonnais, 1981). By interpreting the information collected, the nurse can formulate perceptions about the patient and, where possible, get the patient to validate those perceptions. Theories, frameworks, models and principles are used as approaches to data collection (Christensen, 1982). These approaches give direction and guidance to the assessment process. Nursing models such as those described by Roy (1986), Orem (1985) and Roper *et al.* (1986) all provide parameters to aid patient assessment.

As a general rule, care plans in this book base the patient assessment on activities of daily living. The individual patient in most cases is the primary source of data. Other sources used to collect data include:

1. Family and friends.
2. Medical records.
3. Results of diagnostic tests.
4. Nursing records.

Assessment is an ongoing activity, part of the cycle of the nursing process. The assessment is followed by the nurse, or the nurse and the patient, arriving at one or more of the following conclusions:

1. No problem exists and the patient's health state is intact.
2. No problem exists but there is a potential problem.
3. There is a problem but the patient is coping effectively.
4. A problem exists that the patient needs help with handling.
5. A problem exists but needs further assessment.

Problem statements

The problem is a concise statement of the patient's actual or potential health concern. Clarity and conciseness will help to ensure that the plan is communicated among the health carers. A specific and clearly stated problem is more likely to be read and understood than a lengthy paragraph that needs time to read and interpret. Terms that may be useful in stating patient problems include:

Inability to.
Lack of.
Unable to.
Difficulty in.
Potential for risk.
Impairment of.
Alteration in.
Failure to.
Limited.
Insufficient.
Inappropriate.
Reduced.

An example of a lengthy problem statement is 'Albert would like to stop smoking completely but feels that he needs cigarettes to calm him down. He has reduced from 30 to six a day'. This could be restated as 'Patient states failure to stop smoking following initial reduction from 30 to six a day'. The problem statement should also be specific and be patient centred. Complex problems should be broken down into smaller component parts for rational development of outcome

criteria and interventions. For example 'Impairment of mobility related to thromboembolic brain damage' is too broad and general. This could be restated as 'Impaired voluntary movements of right limbs and trunk related to paralysis and spasticity' and 'Impaired postural balance control related to damage to nervous pathways'. If this is done, then specific and appropriate outcome criteria can be developed for each problem in contrast with vague and general goals or objectives, and long lists of interventions. It should be evident from the foregoing statements that the problem statement should be accompanied by the possible cause or causes and contributing factors. The aetiology of the problem will be directly related to the possible interventions that may be prescribed. For example 'Restricted joint movements related to inflamed joints' will necessitate interventions that may not be applicable to the problem 'Restricted joint movements related to hyperactivity of the spinal stretch reflex'. It may be helpful and improve clarity and continuity of care if the problem statement is accompanied by a brief statement of the subjective and objective data that identified it as a problem. For example the problem 'Impaired mobility related to painful swollen knees' would be accompanied by the findings:

1. Unable to extend knees fully.
2. Posture: knees bent, wide base, back bent.
3. States pain in knees is 5 on scale 0–10.

Many documentation systems have only an initial assessment document which is completed on or soon after admission. The continued identification of problems may be facilitated if a format that includes the subjective and objective assessment data for the problem could be recorded. As new problems are identified, they are accompanied by their assessment data. The problem list should reflect the patient's current health state. This entails regular assessment and update of the problem list.

Outcomes

Care planning requires that there be criteria against which the success or otherwise of the nursing interventions can be assessed or measured. Various terms have been used for this activity, including goals, aims and objectives. Unless it is explicitly stated, these terms do not actively facilitate the writing of the goal as the patient's goal but may allow the focus to be the nurses' goals. In this book the term 'expected outcome' (Mayers, 1983) is used throughout to refer to a statement of desired patient behaviours or clinical signs or symptoms that will indicate that the problem is being resolved or prevented. The expected outcome statement, like the problem statement, should be concise and specific and state clearly what patient behaviours or clinical signs and symptoms will represent alleviation of the problem if that is what is appropriate. The expected outcome statement will represent the criteria that are used to evaluate the effect of the nursing interventions. Mayers (1983) identifies four categories of possible patient outcomes:

1. Patients' self-report about what they know or understand, or how they feel about a specific situation or circumstance. This would include what the patient may say about his/her illness and treatment, or plans for the future. It would also include what the patient may say that he/she feels about for example coming into hospital, having an operation or being told his/her diagnosis. These expected outcome statements would usually start with 'Patient states: understanding of barium meal procedure'.

2. The patient's behaviour related to specific situations. This would refer to behaviours or activities that the nurse can observe, for example agitation and restlessness when first admitted to hospital, or an unsatisfactory technique for capillary blood glucose testing. The outcome statement may then start with the word 'Demonstrates', for example 'Demonstrates correct and accurate capillary blood glucose testing' or 'Demonstrates calm and relaxed posture'.

3. The patient's behaviours and symptoms related to the illness or disease process. This is reflected in laboratory and diagnostic tests, the patient's vital signs, and observing behaviours. These expected outcome statements usually reflect a desire to return to some stated 'norm' or baseline, for example 'Blood glucose values within the limits 3.5–5.0 mmol/litre'. This may also include patient's self report, for example 'Patient states a reduction in pain felt from 6 to 0 on pain scale within 45 min' or 'Respiratory rate reduced from 40 to 20/min within 2 hours'.

4. Expected outcome statements may be related to the patient's environment and would include all aspects which are of significance including family and significant others.

These four categories provide a general framework for possible ways of thinking how to write outcome statements that are patient oriented. However, there is considerable overlap between categories, and it may be less confusing to think of patient outcomes as what patients do and say and how they feel, and clinical manifestations that reflect the patient's health status. There may be combinations of these types of outcome, for example the problem 'Knowledge deficit related to diabetic self-management'. The expected outcomes will be a combination of what the patient says (knowledge about insulin overdose), what the patient demonstrates (correct examination of the feet) and physiological parameters (blood glucose values). Each expected outcome statement should include checking intervals for evaluation. There is little research evidence at present that will help nurses to make predictions about the rate that outcomes for various

problems will be achieved. However, it is important that nurses start to make these predictions, and to record in the evaluation the outcome. This is then a systematic record that may be used in future research to identify realistic outcomes and successful interventions. Where possible, the expected outcome should always be discussed and agreed with the patient and family. Research by Horsley (1982) has shown that collaboration with patients can lead to more effective attainment of goals and improved patient satisfaction.

Interventions

The nursing interventions are selected to help to alleviate the identified problem, and to move the patient towards meeting the stated expected outcomes. The intention is usually to direct the intervention towards altering or alleviating the cause or causes of the problem. This is not always possible, and it is then appropriate to direct the intervention to changing or treating the results or signs and symptoms of the problem. For example 'Impaired mobility related to damage to nervous pathways' will not enable interventions to be directed towards the cause (the damage to nervous pathways), and in this case the interventions will be related to the manifestations of that damage—paralysed limbs and increasing spasticity. However, the problem 'Impaired mobility related to painful knee joints' does enable the intervention to be aimed at the cause of the problem—

reduction or removal of the pain.

In this book the sections entitled 'Rationale' provide the research base for the interventions where this is available. Many interventions prescribed and carried out by nurses and other health care providers do not have an apparent research base. Some are 'tried-and-tested' remedies which seem to work, and some may be based on nothing more than 'folklore'. Some nurses have started to try to identify valid interventions for frequently occurring patient problems (Haller *et al.*, 1979; Bulechek and McCloskey, 1985), and doubtless this will continue to take place in the future. Interventions may not always represent independent nursing activities but may be in collaboration with, or dependent upon, other health care providers such as therapists and doctors.

Evaluation

The expected outcomes which are stated following the assessment and problem identification act as the criteria against which to judge the success of the nursing interventions. The evaluation may be written as the patient's actual outcome in relation

to the interventions prescribed. The outcome statement should be written using the criteria in the expected outcome statement as a guide. For example, if the expected outcome is 'Pressure sore to decrease in size from 45 mm to 40 mm' and this is reviewed at

5-day intervals, then the evaluation or actual outcome statement should state the new measurement and whether or not this is a reduction in size. If the expected outcome was written so as to reflect the patient's statement or behaviour, or the environmental situation, then the actual outcome statement can be written in the same way. The actual or observed patient responses to care are factual statements which, when compared with the expected outcome statement, give a fairly clear indication of the success or failure of the prescribed nursing interventions. Evaluation may have several outcomes:

1. The expected outcomes have been achieved by the patient and the problem has been resolved.
2. The expected outcomes have been achieved by the patient but the problem needs to be monitored further.
3. The expected outcomes have not been realised and so the situation needs to be reassessed:
   a. Was the problem identified the correct one?
   b. Is the cause of the problem still the same?
   c. Are the contributing factors still the same?
   d. Was the problem properly assessed in the first place?
   e. Were the best or correct interventions selected?
   f. Were the interventions consistently implemented?
   g. Were the expected outcomes realistic or appropriate?
   h. Has there been sufficient time to achieve the outcomes?

As was stated earlier, careful recording of actual outcomes in relation to prescribed interventions will provide a rich source of data for researchers to analyse and identify effective and ineffective interventions which may then be subjected to further evaluation.

The nursing process or problem-solving approach, it is argued by Henderson (1982), is not the only approach in nursing. Henderson (1982) is critical of the view that logical deduction is the only way to solve problems and puts a case for the validity of intuitive judgement derived from clinical knowledge as a mode of problem solving which is of equal value to nurses. There is evidence that the more experienced expert nurse is able to grasp the intricacies of a clinical situation rapidly and can sort out relevant from irrelevant information with a well-developed perceptual awareness (Benner, 1984). These nurses are distinguished from the beginner who must rely on a deliberate analytical method to build a clinical picture from isolated pieces of information. Therefore, it becomes important that a systematic framework such as the nursing process is used by nurses and that it is recognised that the nurse's experience and ability will determine how it is used. There is evidence that nurses may be collecting assessment data but for several reasons are failing to examine relationships within the data and so often make poor judgements or do not arrive at appropriate conclusions (Field, 1983). There may therefore be a special need for nurses to be taught how to analyse and interpret assessment data. Therefore, throughout this book, each care plan involves the reader in some interpretation of the assessment data to identify further problems not included in the main care plan. In addition, the reader is also asked to think about other interventions and evaluation criteria which may be relevant to problems already identified. All the care plans relate to 'real' patients. Answers to reader questions are printed on a separate page. All possible problems are not included in the care plans; so it is hoped that the reader will go on to expand the plans and that they are used as teaching tools in wards and classrooms.

References

Benner, P. (1984). *From Novice to Expert*, Addison-Wesley, Menlo Park, California.

Bourbonnais, F. (1981). Pain assessment: development of a tool for the nurse and patient. *Journal of Advanced Nursing*, 6, 277–282.

Bulechek, G. M., and McCloskey, J. C. (1985). *Nursing Interventions. Treatments for Nursing Diagnoses*. W. B. Saunders, Philadelphia, Pennsylvania.

Christensen, P. (1982). Nursing Assessment: data collection of the individual patient. In: Griffith, J. W., and Christensen, P. J. (eds), *Nursing Process. Application of Theories, frameworks, and models*, C. V. Mosby, St Louis, Missouri.

Field, P. A. (1983). An ethnography: four public health nurses' perceptions of nursing. *Journal of Advanced Nursing*, 8, 3–12.

Haller, K. B., Reynolds, M. A., and Horsley, J. A. (1979). Developing research based innovation protocols: process criteria, and issues. *Research in Nursing and Health*, 2, 45–51.

Henderson, V. (1982). The nursing process—is the title right? *Journal of Advanced Nursing*, 7, 103–116.

Horsley, J. A. (1982). Mutual goal setting in patient care. *Conduct and Utilisation of Research in Nursing Project, Michigan Nurses Association*, Grune and Stratton, New York.

Mayers, M. (1983). *A Systematic Approach to the Nursing Care Plan*, Appleton Century Crofts, Norwalk, Connecticut.

Orem, D. (1985). *Nursing: Concepts of Practice*, McGraw-Hill, New York.

Roper, N., Logan, W. W., and Tierney, A. J. (1986). *The Elements of Nursing*, Churchill Livingstone, Edinburgh.

Roy, C. (1986). *Introduction to Nursing, an adaptation model*, Prentice-Hall, Englewood Cliffs, New Jersey.

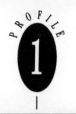

PROFILE

1

Alison Jesson

Rehabilitation after a myocardial infarction:

Health education and counselling for long-term recovery

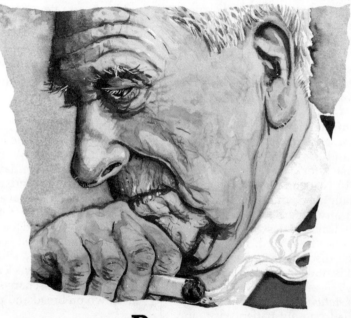

Patients who experience a myocardial infarction often feel helpless, out of control and scared of the future. However, with careful assessment and planning, they can be encouraged to view the experience as a signal for a new start in life. Three problems are outlined, together with causes and expected outcomes, relating to health education and rehabilitation. Further questions are posed; the answers to these are at the end of the chapter.

Patient profile

Geoge Mead was admitted to hospital in mid-May after experiencing severe chest pains. After he had arrived by ambulance in the accident and emergency department, he suffered a cardiac arrest. Electrocardiogram (ECG) and blood enzymes confirmed an anterior myocardial infarct. He made an uneventful recovery and was discharged to stay with his daughter after 8 days. Before discharge, he was assessed by the cardiac counsellor nurse, who felt that he was very anxious about going home and would need continuing support and health education. The recommendation was that he attend an out-patient cardiac rehabilitation programme, consisting of exercise training, relaxation and group discussions.

This assessment was done at the first session, 3 weeks post-discharge.

Assessment information
Biographical and social information
George is 66 and has been retired from the printing industry for a year. He has been divorced for 15 years and lives on his own. He has a daughter who has two small children, and an unmarried son. Both live about 8 miles away. He describes himself as being lonely since he retired. He has spent 2 weeks since discharge staying with his daughter and is now on his own at home.

Current health status
George has had one out-patient visit since discharge when he performed an exercise ECG. This was negative (that is he had no symptoms, nor was there any evidence of ischaemia as he walked on a moving treadmill, attached to an ECG). He has continued to take tab. atenolol 100 mg (a beta blocker) which he took before his heart attack to control hypertension. He says he has lost all his confidence: 'It's silly, but I'm scared to go out of the house, especially after dark.'

Assessment
Communicating
George is pleased to see the familiar face of the cardiac counsellor nurse. He appears nervous, his eyes roam around the room, and he continually shifts his body position. He asks frequent questions about whether or not he is doing the right thing. 'What if I have another attack?'

Circulation and breathing
George's blood pressure is 140/90 mmHg and his heart rate is 65/min and regular. He feels physically well, but tired. He has reduced his smoking from 30 a day before the attack to six or seven a day. He smokes more in the evening. 'I just don't seem to be able to stop. I need them to calm me down.'

Eating and drinking
George weighs 80.7 kg (12 stone 10 lb) and is 5 ft 8 in (1.73 m) tall. He feels that he is about a stone overweight. While he was working, his main meal of the day was in the works canteen. Now he tends to eat convenience and tinned food. An average day's food intake consists of the following. Breakfast: fried bacon, eggs and toast. Lunch: meat pie, potatoes and tinned vegetables. Supper: sausages or a chop, with chips. He drinks 6–7 pints of beer a week and likes cakes and biscuits. Since discharge, he claims to have cut down on bread and potatoes!

Working and playing
Before his heart attack, George was very slowly beginning to make lifestyle changes following retirement. However, he has made few new friends and has few hobbies. He enjoys music, driving to the country and swimming occasionally. Since his divorce, he has had one long-term relationship with another woman, but it ended abruptly, and George feels that he is to blame for this. Since his heart attack, he has hardly ventured outside unaccompanied, but he is keen to get back to driving his car.

Problems, expected outcomes, and interventions

Problem 1

George would like to stop smoking completely but feels that he needs cigarettes to calm him down. He has reduced from 30 to six a day.

Cause

Smoking produces a physical, psychological and social dependency (Beals, 1984).

Expected outcomes

1. That George will understand the importance of stopping smoking.
2. That he will decide a target date by which he will have stopped, and find other methods of relieving tension.

Interventions

1. Explain to George that stopping smoking will reduce the risk of further heart attacks (Mulcahy *et al.*, 1977).
2. Ask George to make a note of every time that he has a cigarette, and his reasons for it (for example thoughts, feelings and events).
3. Teach him relaxation techniques, and provide support at the rehabilitation class.

Question 1

On a separate piece of paper, outline some of the effects of smoking on the body and as many methods of smoking cessation as you can.

Problem 2

Anxiety and fear of leaving home after a heart attack.

Causes

A myocardial infarction, especially one involving a cardiac arrest, is a devastating psychological experience. Inadequate preparation for discharge, and lack of continued support can greatly prolong recovery time (Wilson-Barnett, 1979).

Expected outcomes

1. That George will feel able to share his feelings of anxiety with the group.
2. That he will feel increasingly confident of going out of the house alone.

Interventions

1. Help George to feel part of the group and encourage him to share his feelings.
2. Explain the common reactions to a heart attack (anxiety and depression), and draw on other group members to support this.

Question 2

What other interventions could be used to reduce his anxiety levels and increase his confidence?

Problem 3

George is overweight (14 lb).

Cause
George's diet is high in fat and sugar and lacking in fibre and fresh vegetables.

Expected outcomes
1. That George will understand how to re-organise his diet and will feel motivated to lose weight.
2. That he will set a target date for himself by which time he will have lost 14 lb.

Interventions
1. George will be given an information booklet about which foods he should eat and which to avoid.
2. He will fill in a weekly weight chart and discuss any difficulties with the group.

Question 3

What may be another cause of being overweight in this patient?

Rationale

There are many risk factors associated with myocardial infarction and it is often difficult to identify one sole cause. Some factors such as heredity or diabetes are not possible to change, but others such as smoking, obesity and hypertension are amenable to intervention, and there is evidence that further attacks can be prevented (Mulcahy *et al.*, 1977).

It is important for George to feel that he is back in control of his life after the attack, and a rehabilitation programme can contribute to this. A World Health Organization (WHO, 1968) working group defined cardiac rehabilitation as 'The sum of activities required to ensure the best possible physical, mental, and social conditions, so the patients may, by their own efforts, regain as normal as possible a place in the community and lead an active and productive life' (Deavin, 1984). The main requirement of a rehabilitation programme is that it should be centred on the whole person, and look at personality, lifestyle and other problems (Wilson-Barnett, 1979; Gloag, 1985).

It is more helpful to George to look at why he smokes and to teach him methods to control the cause and the behaviour than merely to tell him to stop.

Having a myocardial infarction can be a devastating psychological experience. Over two-thirds of patients exhibit some evidence of emotional upset, such as anxiety about the future, fear of being alone, poor sleep and so on, which may become severe. If steps are not taken to relieve these symptoms, they may persist for a year or more (Cay, 1984). Adequate preparation for discharge, and supportive counselling both pre- and post-discharge to patient and spouse, can prevent unnecessary invalidism and enhance self-concept, emotional stability and social independence (Mayou *et al.*, 1978; Naismith, 1979).

Rehabilitation for George will consist of exercise training, learning relaxation techniques, and group discussions. Exercise has been shown not only to improve cardio-vascular efficiency but also to contribute to a sense of well-being (Blackburn, 1983). Exercise needs to be gradually increased and carefully prescribed. Learning relaxation techniques can reduce blood pressure permanently and help coping strategies (Boha-

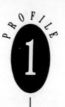

chick, 1984; Patel, 1985). There is also evidence from several trials that a lowering of cholesterol intake and a modification of diet may prevent coronary artery disease. A combination of diet modification and an increase in exercise will result in a lowering of George's weight (ISFC, 1983; Donahoe *et al.*, 1984).

Evaluation

Problem 1

Smoking.

Smoking cessation needs to be evaluated over a period of several weeks, up to and after George's target date for stopping. As he learns to analyse his smoking habits and adopts new methods of relieving tension, he will have more control. After 5 weeks in the group, he had cut his smoking right down to one or two cigarettes every couple of days.

Problem 2

Anxiety on leaving home.

George's contributions to the group and willingness to share his feelings will need to be evaluated over a few weeks. Criteria which could be used to assess increasing confidence include:

1. The number of positive and negative statements that he makes.
2. The number of times that he shares his feelings with the group.

3. The description of his lifestyle and evidence that he is going out more.

After 5 weeks in the group, George joins in the discussions and is thinking about joining an adult education class. He still looks anxious and nervous at times.

Problem 3

Being overweight.

Weight loss may be slow to start with if George is having to reorganise his diet and is trying to stop smoking. Criteria which can be used to assess the likelihood of weight loss include:

1. Is there a consistent weight loss of 1–2 lb per week?
2. Is there an increase in exercise?
3. Is George able to alter his diet pattern and identify healthier foods?

After 5 weeks, George has lost only 3 lb. He has managed to alter his diet pattern but he finds that he often eats a biscuit or sweets instead of having a cigarette.

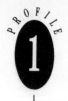

Answers to questions 1, 2 and 3

Problem 1

Question 1

Effects of smoking and methods of cessation.

There is overwhelming evidence to suggest that smoking causes bronchitis, emphysema, cancer of the respiratory tract, coronary artery disease and peripheral vascular disease.

Methods to help stop smoking include (HEC, undated):

1. Behavioural reward, such as buying a present for oneself with the money saved by not smoking.

2. Positive self-talk on the benefits of not smoking, for example increasing health and not smelling of stale tobacco.
3. Making smoking less automatic by keeping matches, cigarettes and ashtray all in separate rooms.
4. For people who have seriously tried to stop on their own, help may also be obtained from nicotine chewing gum, hypnosis, acupuncture and self-help groups.

Problem 2

Question 2

Anxiety levels may be reduced by:

1. Teaching relaxation or meditation techniques with the help of cassette tapes which can be used at home.

2. Rating the causes of anxiety on a scale 1–10 and using problem-solving methods and goal setting to solve some of them.
3. Teaching assertion techniques.

Problem 3

Question 3

Another cause of being overweight may be lack of exercise.

A planned programme of increasing moderate exercise has been shown to reduce weight and to improve self-image and fitness (Naismith, 1979; Donahoe *et al.*, 1984).

References

Beals, A. (1984). The lure of the weed. *Nursing Mirror*, **159**, 8, suppl., XII–XVI.

Blackburn, H. (1983). Physical activity and coronary heart disease: a brief update and population view. *Journal of Cardiac Rehabilitation*, **3**, 101–111.

Bohachick, P. (1984). Progressive relaxation training cardiac rehabilitation. *Nursing Research*, **33**, 283–287.

Cay, E. L. (1984). Psychological problems in patients after myocardial infarction. *Advanced Cardiology*, **29**, 108–112.

Deavin, J. (1984). Rehabilitation following myocardial infarction. *Nursing*, **25**, 740–742.

Donahoe, C., Darria, H., Kirschenbaum, D., and Keese, R. (1984). Metabolic consequences of dieting and exercise in the treatment of obesity. *Journal of Consulting and Clinical Psychology*, **52**(5), 827–836.

Gloag, D. (1985). Rehabilitation of patients with cardiac conditions. *British Medical Journal*, **290**(6468), 617–620.

HEC (undated). *So You Want to Stop Smoking*, Health Education Council, London.

ISFC (1983). *Myocardial Infarction: How to Prevent, How to Rehabilitate*, International Society and Federation of Cardiology.

Mayou, R., Foster, A., and Williamson, B. (1978). The psychological and social effects of myocardial infarction on wives. *British Medical Journal*, **1**(6113), 699–701.

Mulcahy, R., Hickey, N., Graham, I., and Macairt, J. (1977). Factors affecting the five-year survival rate of men following acute coronary disease. *American Heart Journal*, **93**(5), 556–559.

Naismith, L. (1979). Psychological rehabilitation after myocardial infarction. *British Medical Journal*, **1**(6160), 439–446.

Patel, C. (1985). Trial of relaxation in reducing coronary risk: four years' follow-up. *British Medical Journal*, **290**(6475), 1103–1106.

Wilson-Barnett, J. (1979). A review into the research into the experience of patients suffering from coronary thrombosis. *International Journal of Nursing Studies*, **16**, 183–198.

WHO (1968). *Program for Physical Rehabilitation of Patients with Acute Myocardial Infarction*, World Health Organization, Geneva.

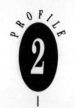

Lynn Batehup

Helping a patient to understand diabetes:

Teaching plan to promote an independent lifestyle

George Campford was admitted to hospital after metabolic control of his diabetes had not been achieved while he was being treated as an outpatient. He is frustrated and appears not to understand fully the management of his condition. Some nursing problems are outlined, together with their expected outcomes and interventions. The organisation of a teaching programme for Mr Campford and ideas on how to ensure that safe blood glucose levels are maintained for him are required; the answers appear at the end of the chapter.

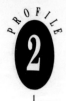

Patient profile

Mr George Campford, aged 53, was admitted for control of diabetes after having been diagnosed as having the condition 2 months previously. At first, his diabetes was regarded as being non-insulin dependent but, as metabolic control was not achieved, insulin was started in the outpatient department, supervised by a hospital-attached diabetic nurse specialist.

In the event, metabolic control was still not achieved, and Mr Campford was admitted to hospital.

Assessment information
Biographical and social information
George Campford is married with two grown-up children who are married and live away from home. He lives with his wife in his own three-bedroom terraced house in a road opposite the hospital. Mrs Campford works as a junior manager in a large retail firm in the centre of London, and her job is quite demanding. Mr Campford is a self-employed motor cycle courier and has been in this job for 5 years.

Current health status
At the moment, Mr Campford feels unwell and 'under par—mainly because of my high blood sugar'. However, when this problem of poor control is sorted out, he feels confident that life will go on as before—with the exception that 'the job of motor cycle courier will have to go'. He is frustrated and impatient that the control of his blood sugar is taking so long. He feels that it should have been cleared up by now and says that his wife is urging him to 'go privately' in order to get things done more quickly.

Mrs Campford is worried about her husband's condition, but she is sure that eventually he will adapt to having diabetes.

A year ago, Mr Campford was admitted to hospital with bleeding oesophageal varices and found to have alcoholic cirrhosis. Following treatment for the varices, there has been no further bleeding. He continues to have some degree of liver enlargement.

Assessment
Eating and drinking
Mr Campford has lost 7 kg over the last 3 months; he now weighs 65 kg. He is 5 ft 8 in tall.

The dietary assessment indicates that his daily total energy intake is in the region of 2700 kcal. With Mr Campford's agreement, a diet consisting of 230 g of carbohydrate, 2500 kcal, high fibre low fat, was started. On admission, he was taking Mixtard insulin 45 units before breakfast and 40 units before the evening meal. Blood glucose levels in excess of 22 mmol/litre were the consistent finding. Polydipsia had been present before diagnosis, but this was not now a problem.

Alcohol intake before September 1984 had been about a bottle of whisky over 2–3 days, or 3–4 pints of beer daily. Since the bleeding varices last year, Mr Campford states that he has not taken any alcohol, and Mrs Campford substantiates this information. Random blood alcohol levels are negative.

The current insulin regime is short-acting Humulin insulin twice daily, and intermediate-acting insulin once daily.

Eliminating
Polyuria had been a problem, but this was now not so. Mr Campford had been testing his own urine with Ketodiastix. He has now stopped because capillary blood is used for blood glucose estimations. Ketonuria is not present.

Communicating
Understanding the disease Mr Campford was given booklets to read when at home and seems to have quite a high level of understanding. On specific questioning, however, he shows that he has misconceptions in several areas. He is a very talkative extrovert individual who appears confident and knowledgeable.
Barriers to learning English is Mr Campford's first language. He left school at 15 and since then has read widely. He has many

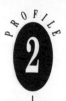

interests and appears intelligent and motivated (in fact, excessive confidence may be a barrier). At present, he is having difficulty with his vision, specifically blurring and fuzziness.

Working and playing
Mr Campford has always been self-employed in various types of work. At present, he is a motor cycle courier in central London. 'It is a strenuous and exhausting job', but he gets a good salary. He has not worked for the past 3 months and says that, although he is not overly worried about money, he hopes to get back to work as soon as possible. He is hoping to find a different job—he has decided that he should 'settle down' and get something more appropriate to his age (there are only two other couriers in London older than he

is). For recreation, Mr Campford and his wife enjoy walking, reading and going to the theatre or to see a film. He does not take part in any sports—he states that his job is sport enough.

Sleeping
Mr Campford usually sleeps about 7 hours a night. At present, he is getting 11–12 hours and also sleeps for periods throughout the day. He puts this down to high blood sugar— he feels drowsy and has a 'muzzy' head when his blood sugar is elevated. In the morning, he wakes with a headache.

Personal hygiene
As Mr Campford lives just outside the hospital, he walks home alone for a shower, shave and change of clothes daily.

Problems, expected outcomes, and interventions

Problem 1

Failure to maintain safe blood glucose levels, probably related to pancreatic insufficiency, secondary to alcoholic liver disease. Replacement with exogenous insulin is not resulting in the effective control of Mr Campford's blood sugar.

Cause 1
Inadequate replacement levels of insulin. The medical staff are increasing dosage according to the fasting and pre-prandial blood glucose levels.

Expected outcome
Fasting blood glucose values of less than 7 mmol/litre, and post-prandial values of less than 10 mmol/litre.

Intervention
In this instance, intervention relates to the medical management—interpreting blood glucose records and prescription of insulin

dose. Nursing intervention would include ensuring correct dosage and timing of insulin, and monitoring its effects.

Cause 2
Ineffective self-management of diet, blood glucose monitoring and insulin administration.

Expected outcome
Improved and effective skills for self-management of diabetes, as reflected in more normal blood glucose values fasting and after meals.

Interventions
Devise a teaching plan which may include the following topics (Marks, 1983):

1. What is diabetes, and what causes it?
2. How is diabetes controlled?
3. What is meant by a diabetic diet?

4. Urine testing and blood testing. How and why?
5. Equipment: how to use it, and look after it.
6. Foot care.
7. What are the early complications? The later complications?
8. How will diabetes affect me at work, and my lifestyle in general?

Question 1

Can you suggest which factors it would be important to assess before starting a teaching programme such as this?

Question 2

On a separate sheet of paper, can you suggest two other causes for failure to maintain safe blood glucose levels, with their expected outcomes and interventions?

Problem 2

Mr Campford has unrealistic expectations for dramatic and rapid recovery at this early stage of diagnosis and treatment.

Cause
His previous illness experience related to treatment of oesophageal varices was an emergency and quickly dealt with. The recovery was also prompt and straightforward.

Expected outcome
Mr Campford should be able to state the differences between the illness experienced 1 year ago, and the present problem of establishing stability in blood glucose control and lifestyle.

Intervention
It is to be expected that an effective diabetic teaching programme will highlight the delicate balance that has to be achieved between diet, insulin and activity. However, this requires more prolonged and intense activity on the part of the patient and health carers.

Question 3

On a separate sheet of paper, can you suggest one other cause for Mr Campford's unrealistic expectations for his recovery?

Rationale

Diabetes is a condition in which self-management is uniquely important; therefore it is essential that diabetics have high levels of skill and knowledge about managing the condition.

In patients whose regime is carefully planned to co-ordinate meals, exercise and other activities with the hypothetical action of injected insulin, variations in insulin absorption and sensitivity become major determinants of fluctuations in the blood glucose levels (Binder *et al.*, 1984). Reproducible technique is important and should be aimed at placing the depot of insulin into the subcutaneous tissues (Lauritzen *et al.*, 1982). This ensures consistent absorption.

Accuracy in drawing up insulin by diabetic patients has been found to be relatively low (Wright *et al.*, 1982) and, in addition, varying 'dead space' of syringes has been found to be responsible for causing errors in insulin dose of up to 10 units (Skodda *et al.*, 1983). Also of importance are the regional differences in absorption rates, with absorption slowing in both diabetics and healthy individuals as one moves from the abdomen to the arm, with the slowest being in the thigh (Koivisto and Felig, 1980). These findings suggest that daily random site rotation can produce erratic insulin levels. It is probably better to stay within one area until all available sites have been used before moving to another area. It is a safe approach not to use the same areas more often than once every 4–6 weeks (Thatcher, 1985). There is also evidence that exercise and massage of the injected limb after injecting short-acting insulin may increase the rate of insulin absorption (Binder *et al.*, 1984).

Self-monitoring of blood glucose has enabled the diabetic patient to evaluate effects of diet, exercise and stress on diabetic control. Capillary blood letting is made more acceptable and less painful by the development of spring-loaded needle holders, with the ability to vary the depth of penetration for various skin thicknesses. Recommended puncture areas are the sides of the finger tips, where there are fewer nerve endings and a rich capillary bed for more painless and successful blood letting. Puncture sites can be prepared with soap and water (Valenta, 1983). Some glucose oxidase strips, for example BM-Test Glycaemie (Boehringer Mannheim), do not require a meter for assessment. Their effects on diabetic control have not been clearly established, but some studies have shown that diabetics can use them accurately (Rayman *et al.*, 1984).

Dietary control is used in combination with exercise and medication to maintain blood glucose levels at near normal physiological range. Long-term vascular complications in diabetics may be related to dietary practice via both the degree of glycaemic control and the composition of the diet in respect of the fat, carbohydrate and fibre intake (Nutrition Sub-Committee of the Medical Advisory Committee to the British Diabetic Association, 1982a). Each diabetic requires dietary advice given on an individual basis, related to total energy requirements with the former practice of simple set 'diet sheets' now inadequate. Individual advice and education should be given by a qualified dietitian and should incorporate the recent British Diabetic Association recommendations of increased complex carbohydrate and less fat (Nutrition Sub-Committee of the Medical Advisory Committee to the British Diabetic Association, 1982b).

The role of psychological as well as physical stress in raising blood sugar should not be underestimated. Through the hypothalamic–pituitary–adrenal axis, gluconeogenesis and glycogenolysis is stimulated with an increase in available glucose in all parts of the body (Guyton, 1981). Stress can be reduced through relaxation techniques, and exercise, even when mild, can be beneficial in lowering negative effects of stress (Guthrie and Guthrie, 1982).

Except when the individual is in with, for example, an infection, or following a surgical operation, appropriate exercise can help with maintenance of physiological levels of blood glucose.

Hypoglycaemia results from inadequate amounts of circulating glucose to keep pace with the rate of glucose use. Peripheral tissues can use fats for energy if insufficient glucose is available, but the brain relies on glucose for its source of fuel. Hypoglycaemia can result from too much insulin relative to food intake and/or exercise. This imbalance may be caused by changing of the insulin dose by the patient or doctor, a visual impairment causing an inaccurate dose to be administered, a reduced need for insulin because of lowered calorie intake, skipping or delaying meals, weight loss or an increase in the amount of exercise without adequate food intake (Harmon Moorman, 1983). The use of alcohol

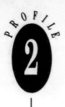

in the patient taking insulin may block gluco-neogenesis and produce severe hypogly-caemia if the patient has not eaten for a while (Cavalier, 1980).

Hyperglycaemia arises when the lack of insulin prevents the utilisation of glucose by almost all tissues of the body, and its accumulation in the bloodstream. Apart from insufficient insulin, the causes of hyper-glycaemia in diabetic patients may be related to excessive food intake or eating the wrong kinds of food, decreased activity levels in relation to food intake, and emotional stress and illness or infection. When ill, patients frequently reduce their food intake and also their insulin dosage out of fear of hypogly-caemia; yet the stress of illness raises the blood glucose level and increases the need for insulin despite any reduction in food intake. It is important, therefore, that the patient is instructed in the management of diabetes during illness. Advice could include such facts as the need to take the usual dose of insulin, to test urine or blood for sugar at least four times a day and to test urine for ketones; if additional insulin is required, the patient should be advised to take short-acting insulin, to rest and keep warm, to take some form of fluid each hour and, if unable to eat the usual diet, to substitute semiliquid foods for the carbohydrate content and to call the doctor if the illness becomes prolonged (Bovington et al., 1983).

Evaluation

The following criteria can be used to evaluate the patient's self-management abilities.

Knowledge of diabetes

1. Is the patient able to understand what diabetes is and that it is present for his lifetime? Does the family understand this?
2. What emotions and feelings are the patient and family showing?
3. What expectations do the patient and family have for future lifestyle changes?

Self-management for insulin controlled patients

1. Is the patient able to understand the need for daily insulin or oral hypoglycaemic drug?
2. Is the patient able to understand the in-sulin action and side-effects?
3. Is the patient able to prepare and ad-minister accurate doses of insulin, to understand the concepts of cleanliness and asepsis where appropriate, and to store insulin, syringes and needles correctly?
4. Is the patient able to:
   a. Test urine or blood efficiently and accurately?
   b. Keep a record of urine or blood glucose values, and insulin dose?
   c. Comment why the glucose level was too high or too low?
   d. Record urinary ketones when glucose is high?
5. a. Is patient rotating injection sites in a planned fashion?
   b. Is fatty change present at injection sites?
6. a. Is patient having hypoglycaemic episodes? If so, how often, and at what time of day?
   b. How does he manage these episodes? How much insulin is being taken, and at what time of day?
   c. Is he adjusting the insulin dose? Under what circumstances? By how much?
7. a. Is patient having symptoms of hyper-glycaemia?
   b. Does blood glucose record show good or poor control?
   c. Is the patient complaining of night sweats or early morning headaches?
8. a. Is the patient keeping to the recom-mended diet?
   b. Are meals and snacks taken at the times corresponding to peak insulin action?

c. Is the patient able to maintain lifestyle?

9. a. Is patient able to understand effects of activity and exercise on blood glucose control?
   b. Has activity pattern changed?
10. Has the patient had skin rashes or stomach upsets since starting insulin?
11. Is the patient able to understand and carry out foot and skin care?

Knowledge of hyperglycaemia

1. How would you know if your blood glucose was getting too high?
2. What might cause you to have too much sugar in your blood?
3. What would you do if you have signs of high blood sugar?

4. Why is it important to prevent blood sugar from getting too high?
5. What would you do to manage your diabetic state when ill?
6. What would you do if you are ill for more than 24 hours?

Knowledge of hypoglycaemia

1. How would you know if your blood sugar was too low?
2. What might cause you to have too little sugar in your blood?
3. What would you do if you have signs of a low blood sugar?
4. Why is it important to prevent blood sugar from getting too low?

Answers to questions 1, 2 and 3

Problem 1

Question 1

Before beginning a teaching programme, it is important to consider the patient's readiness to learn both emotional readiness or motivation, and experiential readiness which includes the individual's background or experiences, skills and attitudes. It is also necessary to consider the special senses, including vision, hearing, touch and colour vision. Physical condition also affects learning ability, in this case fluctuating blood glucose levels.

Teaching methods that provide practice, a great deal of feedback, reinforcement and correction, and those that require patient participation during learning are more likely to be successful.

Problem 1

Question 2

Two other causes of failure to maintain safe blood glucose levels might include the following.

Cause 1
Psychological stress related to the onset of diabetes.

Expected outcome
Mr Campford should be able to demonstrate an understanding that emotional upsets, anxiety, fear or anticipation that diabetes will have an adverse effect on lifestyle can affect blood glucose control.

Intervention
The stress of illness and everyday life can be managed if both the patient and the nurse are aware of the effects of stress upon diabetic control. The patient's fears and anxieties about having to carry out the daily tasks of urine or blood testing, giving insulin and eating correctly, and also knowledge about future implications of the disease, can be incomplete and inaccurate. This can cause high levels of stress and anxiety and adversely affect control. The role of the nurse is to help the patient to identify worries and gaps in knowledge and skills and to help him to do something to correct it. Some patients are helped by talking to other diabetic persons, and by support groups such as the British Diabetic Association.

Cause 2
Mr Campford's visual impairment (blurring of vision) may cause him to draw up an inaccurate insulin dose.

Expected outcome
Mr Campford should be able to draw up and give himself the prescribed insulin dose accurately.

Intervention
It should be acceptable for the nurse to give some help in supervising the insulin injection while Mr Campford's vision is blurred. In this instance, Mr Campford did feel somewhat resentful that he was being supervised and felt that he was not trusted, but it should be possible to overcome this problem with tactful discussion with him.

Problem 2

Question 3

The other reason for Mr Campford's unrealistic expectations for his recovery is as follows.

Cause
Some degree of denial of the chronic nature of diabetes. Mr Campford sees himself and his state of health as vigorous and invincible, despite having knowledge of his relatively severe liver disease. He therefore expects to recover quickly.

Expected outcome
Mr Campford should maintain high self-esteem while describing accurate knowledge of current or potential health problems. It is hoped that he will demonstrate by verbal statement some degree of acceptance of the long-term characteristics of diabetes.

Intervention
As with Problem 1, Cause 1, the teaching programme should be helping Mr Campford to deal with and adapt to the condition. Continuous self-management by the patient is crucial for good diabetic control. Mr Campford needs to be able to make decisions and to take actions in order to maintain his usual lifestyle. The family members, especially the spouse, feel the same worries and emotions as the patient. The nurse should consider the family role in self-management and be aware of the influence that this has on the patient.

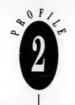

PROFILE
2

References

Binder, C., Lauritzen, T., Faber, O., and Pramming, S. (1984). Diabetes care. *Insulin Pharmacokinetics*, **7** (2) 188–199.

Bovington, N. M., Enzenauer Spies, M., and Troy, P. J. (1983). Management of the patient with diabetes mellitus during surgery and illness. *Nursing Clinics of North America*, **18** (4) 661–671.

Cavalier, J. P. (1980). Crucial decisions in diabetic emergencies. *Registered Nurse*, **43**, 32.

Guthrie, D. W., and Guthrie, R. A. (1982). *Nursing Management of Diabetes Mellitus*, C. V. Mosby, St Louis, Missouri.

Guyton, A. C. (1981). *Textbook of Medical Physiology*, W. B. Saunders, Philadelphia, Pennsylvania.

Harmon Moorman, N. (1983). Acute complications of hyperglycaemia and hypoglycaemia. *Nursing Clinics of North America*, **18** (4) 707–719.

Koivisto, V. A., and Felig, P. (1980). Alterations in insulin absorption and in blood glucose control associated with varying insulin injection sites in diabetic patients. *Annals of Internal Medicine*, **92**, 59–61.

Lauritzen, T., Pramming, S., Gale, E. A. M., Deckert, T., and Binder, C. (1982). Absorption of isophane insulin and its clinical implications. *British Medical Journal*, **285**, 159–162.

Marks, C. (1983). Teaching the diabetic patient. In: Wilson-Barnett, J. (ed), *Patient Teaching*, Churchill Livingstone, Edinburgh.

Nutrition Sub-Committee of the Medical Advisory Committee of the British Diabetic Association (1982a). The role of the dietitian in the management of the diabetic. *Human Nutrition: Applied Nutrition,* **36A**, 395–400.

Nutrition Sub-Committee of the Medical Advisory Committee to the British Diabetic Association (1982b). Dietary recommendations for diabetics in the 1980s. A policy statement by the British Diabetic Association. *Human Nutrition: Applied Nutrition*, **36A**, 138–141.

Rayman, G., Dorrington-Ward, P., Ellwood-Russell, M., and Wise, P. (1984). Simple, economical and effective home blood glucose monitoring. *The Practitioner*, **228**, 191–194.

Skodda, H., Warzecha, P., Mulhauser, I., Kemmer, F. W., and Jorgens, V. (1983). The quality of different insulin syringes. *Diabetologia*, **25**, 194.

Thatcher, G. (1985). Insulin injections. The case against random rotation. *American Journal of Nursing*, **6**, 690–692.

Valenta, C. L. (1983). Urine testing and home blood glucose monitoring. *Nursing Clinics of North America*, **18** (4), 645–670.

Wright, S., Morris, J. T., and Hartog, M. (1982). The accuracy of drawing up insulin by insulin-treated diabetics. *Diabetes Metabolism*, **8**, 7–8.

PROFILE
3

Val Thomson

Assisting a mother to establish breastfeeding:

Planning for a happy and successful postnatal period

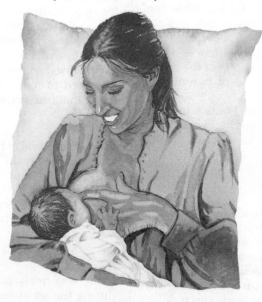

Ruth had been delivered normally
of a healthy son but required help with breastfeeding and in
adapting to motherhood. Some of Ruth's problems are outlined and suggestions are made for assisting her. Further
potential problems need to be identified, together with the
interventions necessary; the answers are at the end of the
chapter.

Patient profile

Ruth is a 26 year old who was admitted to the post-natal ward after having had a normal delivery. Paul, her son, is a healthy infant weighing 3.5 kg. Ruth has chosen to stay in hospital for a few days to establish breastfeeding.

Assessment information

Biographical and social information

Ruth has been married to Frank for 4 years. They have a loving relationship in which they are able to discuss most problems.

Ruth has worked as an interpreter but decided not to return to work after the baby was born, although she was eligible for maternity leave. They are reasonably well off and Ruth has claimed all her allowances.

Ruth's own childhood experiences were good; this will influence her care of the baby. She also attended a course of parentcraft classes.

Both Ruth's mother and Frank's mother will be supportive but might become invasive. The couple also have friends with children.

Current health status

Having had all the childhood illnesses except rubella, Ruth was screened for rubella immunity pre-conceptually and was offered the vaccine, which then conferred immunity.

Her general health is good, but as a routine precaution her blood group and Rhesus (Rh) factor were checked. Although she was Rh negative, she needed no treatment as Frank was found to be Rh negative as well. Her haemoglobin before delivery was 12 g/dl and, as blood loss at delivery was minimal, there is unlikely to be any change in this level.

Ruth had suffered from slight physiological oedema of the legs because of reduced venous return caused by the relaxation of smooth muscle and the pressure of the enlarging uterus on the major veins. Apart from this, she had remained healthy and fit throughout pregnancy.

Assessment

On admission, Ruth was greeted by the ward staff. Information about pregnancy and labour was given.

Her uterus was abdominally palpated and was found to be well contracted. Vaginal loss (lochia) was within normal limits. These observations indicate that the bleeding placental site had achieved haemostasis— contraction of the oblique and circular muscle layer of the uterus acts as a living ligature to the uterine blood vessels.

Eating and drinking

Ruth has a healthy appetite. She had 'eaten for two' during pregnancy and expected to eat well now. She was concerned about hospital food and asked her relatives to bring her supplements to the hospital diet. She was pleased to know that women were encouraged to make their own drinks as she knew that breastfeeding increased thirst.

Sleeping

Towards the end of her pregnancy, Ruth had found difficulty in sleeping and was prepared for interrupted nights when caring for her baby. She did voice some concern, however, as lack of sleep made her irritable and short tempered. She hoped that she might 'catnap' in the day.

Elimination

Urine was freely passed during labour and during the short second stage of labour her bladder and urethra did not sustain any trauma and no problems were expected. She was keen to do exercises to strengthen the pelvic floor muscles as soon as possible. As most pregnant women suffer from a degree of constipation, Ruth was reconciled to this and was confident that normal bowel action would return.

Personal hygiene

Ruth bathed daily at home and intended to continue this while in hospital and also to

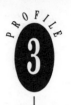

use the bidet regularly throughout the day. Although her perineum was intact, she realised the benefits of cleanliness in reducing uterine infection.

Sexuality

Ruth and Frank had discussed their changing feelings during pregnancy. They hoped that the baby would bring them closer together but had considered the stresses that parenthood might put on their relationship. They were reassured to know that they could resume intercourse as soon as they wished.

Communications

Ruth had not had a chance to formulate a birth plan but felt that she had been able to express her wishes and would be able to

assess her own needs. She had attended parentcraft classes and felt confident in caring for her baby, with support when necessary. However, she was worried about care of Paul's umbilical cord and about the possibility of not being able to perform this task adequately.

Mobility

After delivery, Ruth was tired and wished to rest for a few hours before taking responsiblity for Paul's care. She was aware of the benefits of early mobilisation and decided to do ankle circling exercises while in bed. These exercises reduce the likelihood of thrombosis and also help to resolve any ankle oedema.

Problems, expected outcomes, and interventions

Problem 1

Potential difficulty in establishing adequate lactation.

Causes

Incorrect position of baby at breast; interrupted feeding pattern; psychological reasons.

Expected outcomes

1. Baby's mouth should cover the areola rather than the nipple. This allows correct stripping action of the ducts and the ampullae of the breast.
2. Complete demand breastfeeding, excluding supplements and water.
3. Mother relaxed and confident, allowing normal neurohormonal reflex.

Interventions

1. Be available to support Ruth when Paul wakes for a feed. Assess level of knowl-

edge and add to it, if necessary using a diagram of the correct positioning of the baby at the breast. When Ruth has positioned Paul correctly, describe the factors that indicate this. Make sure that Ruth is in a comfortable position.
2. Explain in acceptable terms the neurohormonal response to sucking, highlighting the supply and demand aspect of breastfeeding. Guide Ruth in assessing the baby's needs. Explain that babies have no need of extra fluids.
3. Maintain continuity of advice and therefore develop Ruth's confidence. Ensure privacy; encourage Ruth to talk to other mums who have breastfed, in order to share their experiences. If Paul is unsettled, it may be necessary for staff to soothe him, allowing Ruth some time to regain her confidence.

Question 1

On a separate sheet of paper, list other psychological problems which might inhibit a woman from successful breastfeeding, particularly in a hospital environment.

Problem 2

Potential infection of the umbilical cord.

Causes
Ruth is unaware of the need for efficient cleaning or has not been encouraged to attend to it; poor technique; she is unwilling to perform the task.

Expected outcome
Clean dry cord separating from umbilicus by process of dry necrosis.

Question 2

On a separate sheet of paper, list the interventions which would prevent this potenial problem.

Problem 3

Potential difficulty in adapting to motherhood.

Causes
Third-day 'blues', depression and anxieties about the change in self-image; lack of confidence in parentcraft abilities; lack of sleep.

Expected outcome
That Ruth has a realistic view of the emotional and psychological changes that may occur and can view such changes in a positive way.

Interventions
1. Provide an environment where Ruth feels free to express her emotions. She can then realise that this is a transitory period and that most women experience these feelings. Also helping her to identify support in her local community.
2. Support and encourage her to care for the baby rather than acting for her.
3. Provide quiet times when she can rest.

Question 3

What support systems might Ruth identify in her community?

Rationale

Pregnancy and the subsequent return to the non-pregnant state are normal physiological events. In the post-natal period, the midwife's role lies in observing the mother's return to her pre-pregnancy state, in promoting health in both mother and baby and in supporting, advising and guiding the mother's care of her baby, occasionally performing some of these tasks herself.

Orem's model of self-care (Pearson, 1986) identifies that areas of need may arise when an otherwise independent individual reaches a life stage cycle such as childbearing or when life changes occur, such as when dependent neonate adapts from intra-uterine to extra-uterine life. Such development self-care needs may be met by enabling the mother to increase her ability in this area and also by enabling the baby's care takers (primarily the mother) to give care to her dependant. In some instances, the need may have to be met directly by the midwife.

A careful appraisal of the mother's perceived needs is necessary in order to plan her subsequent care. The midwife may realise goals either by providing an optimum environment or by supporting, guiding, teaching and in some cases acting for the mother.

In Ruth's case, her perceived needs were met by a combination of helping methods.

In order to establish lactation, a calm peaceful environment in which the mother feels relaxed and confident is essential. Lactation is initiated by the delivery of the placenta. When levels of oestrogen and progesterone fall, their inhibitory effect on prolactin is lost.

The successful establishment of lactation depends on the fact that adequate amounts of prolactin are available. The baby suckling at the mother's breast stimulates the pituitary gland via the hypothalamus to produce prolactin which acts on the acini cells in the alveoli of the breast tissue to produce milk. This milk will not be available for the current feed but, in effect, by sucking, the baby is placing an order for its next feed. If this mechanism is interrupted by offering supplementary feeding or water, especially during the night (studies of prolactin levels show them to be highest at night (Howie, 1985)), then sufficient milk may not subsequently be available.

The correct position of the baby at the breast ensures that he is able to obtain milk without becoming frustrated and/or causing nipple damage (Fisher, 1986). The practice of giving water is unnecessary (DHSS, 1980) as the foremilk contained in the lactiferous ducts is less rich and will satisfy thirst. The other practice of restricting sucking time at the breast in order to protect the nipples also causes the baby to get only foremilk and not the more satisfying hindmilk (Fisher, 1985).

Oxytocin is also necessary to establish lactation; it causes contraction of the alveoli of the breast in order to let down the milk contained therein. Ruth will experience a tingling in her breasts when her baby cries, or even if she thinks of Paul she may leak milk (McNeilly et al., 1983). This action is maintained by suckling at the breast. As the reflex is neurohormonal, an upset can easily disturb its release (Oakley, 1981); Ruth may produce the milk but, if she feels anxious about Paul's feeding or feels embarrassed about exposing her breasts, the let-down reflex will be inhibited, which may worsen the situation.

A supportive environment is essential for learning new skills (Maternity Services Advisory Committee, 1985). Ruth expressed concern about caring for Paul's cord and in this case the midwife may act for the mother. Cord care is not a skill that is necessary for the mother to repeat, once the cord has separated. It can easily be cleaned by the midwife, who will be visiting the baby until separation has occurred. Thus the self-care deficiency is quickly resolved.

The process of adaptation to motherhood is a complex issue; negative feelings are normal but it is essential to allow their expression. Oakley (1981) found that 91% of women thought that motherhood did not

meet their expectations, 84% experienced some kind of depression and the majority noted a degree of marital conflict.

The mood swings of pregnancy are replaced by the classic third-day blues also thought to have a hormonal basis although other compounding factors are normal anxieties about child care capabilities and lack of sleep.

Many health visitors and lay groups have recognised that maternal isolation is a key factor in depression. Post-natal support groups allow free discussion among mothers, where they can share their fears and anxieties so that these are reduced to normal experiences. These support groups also provide a social environment for those who do not have any other contact with mothers and young babies.

Evaluation

Problem 1

Establishment of lactation.

The best indicator of success is a contented baby who settles and sleeps between feeds. However, weight gain is a more tangible evaluation, and Ruth may need this reassurance (Houston, 1981).

While in the midwife's care, Paul should be weighed on a regular basis. After the initial weight loss (maximum, 10% of birth weight on the third day), Paul should show a steady increase to regain his birth weight by the tenth day of life.

Follow-up visits to the well-baby clinic will provide further opportunity to assess growth. This will be recorded on the centile chart.

Ruth did establish a satisfactory breast-feeding routine.

Problem 2

Potential infection of the umbilical cord.

The cord should separate between the seventh and tenth day and certainly before the midwife discharges Paul from her care. Daily observations should be carried out to assess:

1. Healing. The cord should not appear moist or bleeding or have an offensive odour.

2. Correct positioning of the stump outside the nappy. This allows air to circulate.
3. That the surrounding area is clean. There should be no sign of septic spots.

Ruth was reluctant to handle the cord, but separation and healing occurred without any problem.

Problem 3

Potential difficulty in adapting to motherhood.

Motherhood should never be seen in isolation and, in order to assess the process for adaptation, one needs to look at the mother and baby as a unit. Areas of observation should include:

1. How Ruth handles Paul. Whether her actions are merely perfunctory or whether the interaction provides stimulation for both of them.
2. Whether Ruth encourages Frank to participate in Paul's care.
3. Noting whether Ruth appears nervous or tense.
4. Noting how much sleep she is able to have.

Ruth did establish a satisfactory breast-feeding routine.

Answers to questions 1, 2 and 3

Problem 1

Question 1

Other psychological problems which might inhibit successful breastfeeding are:

1. Relatives and staff doubting whether Ruth has adequate breast milk.
2. Staff busy or unable to give enough attention, causing Ruth embarrassment when asking for help.
3. Hospital routine, so that feeding time coincides with Ruth's meal times.
4. Knowing that prepared feeds can be made available instantly.
5. Seeing other mothers bottle feeding.
6. Feeding at night and the fear that the baby is keeping others awake.
7. Not having a fixed feeding routine (Culpin, 1984).

Problem 2

Question 2

Interventions which would prevent infection of the cord are:

1. Talking to Ruth about cord care. Teach her how to clean it if she has not been shown. Assess her level of knowledge and give information to motivate regular attention.
2. Being available at nappy changing time to guide and support Ruth; reassuring her that it does not hurt the baby.
3. Allowing staff to undertake the care of the cord if Ruth is unwilling to do so.

Problem 3

Question 3

Support systems Ruth might identify in her community are:
1. Helpful neighbours and friends willing to babysit.
2. Mother and baby groups.
3. Mother and mother-in-law.
4. National Childbirth Trust post-natal support groups.
5. Health visitor.
6. CRYSIS (Gray, 1986).
7. Association of Breastfeeding Mothers (Beck, 1986).

Useful addresses

CRYSIS: Contact Zita Thornton, 63 Putney Road, Freezywater, Enfield EN3 6NN.

Association of Breastfeeding Mothers: 131 Mayow Rd, Sydenham, London SE26 4HZ.

PROFILE
3

References

Beck, M. (1986). Breastfeeding support group in Taunton. *Midwifes Chronicle*, **99** (1178), 67–68.

Culpin, E. (1984). Expectations of breastfeeding. *Midwives Chronicle*, **97** (1163), 402–403.

DHSS (1980). *Present Day Practice in Infant Feeding*, Department of Health and Social Security, London.

Fisher, C. (1985). How did we go wrong with breastfeeding? *Midwifery*, **1** (1), 48–51.

Fisher, C. (1986). On demand breastfeeding. *Midwife Health Visitor and Community Nurse*, **22** (6), 194–198.

Gray, P. (1986). The constantly crying child. *Midwives Chronicle*, **99** (1180), 108.

Houston, M. (1981). Breastfeeding success or failure. *Journal of Advanced Nursing*, **6** (81), 447–454.

Howie, P. (1985). Breastfeeding—a new understanding. *Midwives Chronicle*, **98** (1170), 184–192.

Maternity Services Advisory Committee (1985). *Maternity Care in Action, Part 3, Care of Mother and Baby*, HMSO, London.

McNeilly, A. S., Robinson, I. C., Houston, M. J. *et al.* (1983). Release of oxytocin and prolactin in response to suckling. *British Medical Journal* **286** (6361), 257–259.

Oakley, A. (1981). *From Here to Maternity*, Penguin, Harmondsworth, Middlesex.

Pearson, A. and Vaughan, B. (1986). *Nursing Models for Practice*, Heinemann, London, p. 69.

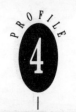
Lynn Batehup

A patient who has had cardiac surgery to relieve unstable angina:

Planning in the acute recovery stage

Coronary vein graft surgery was advised for 51-year-old John to allow him to pursue the most fulfilling lifestyle. Some of the problems that John experienced after transfer from the intensive care unit are outlined and causes, expected outcomes and interventions are detailed. Some further questions are then posed requiring interventions to solve the problems; the answers are provided at the end of the chapter.

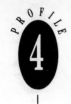

Patient profile

John Manley was admitted to hospital in mid-June for the purpose of investigating his chest pain and because of his shortness of breath. The result was an operation to revascularise his heart muscle using vein grafts.

Assessment information
Biographical and social information
John is 51 years old and has been married to Jean for 27 years. They have two married daughters, who live quite near. John describes his family as 'close' and is obviously proud of them.

Current health status
John had a heart attack in 1984 from which he says that he has fully recovered and resumed his usual job and lifestyle.

Since April of this year, John has been getting increasingly short of breath, at first when doing heavy physical work, and then even when 'I'm not exerting myself'. He continued to do his job, which is very physically demanding, by taking glyceryl trinitrate tablets before heavy work.

In June, John awoke with pains in his arms and chest. This caused him concern and resulted in his visiting his doctor, who referred him to the local hospital, where he was admitted.

In hospital, the pain was relieved only by continuous intravenous infusion of isosorbide dinitrate. John was diagnosed as having 'unstable angina'. This necessitated referral to a cardiac unit, where cardiac catheterisation showed major narrowing and blockage of the important coronary arteries. Following discussion with the surgical team, John decided that coronary vein graft surgery would allow him to pursue the most fulfilling lifestyle.

Assessment
Breathing
John has been getting short of breath after walking about 200 yards. He has no difficulty sleeping on one pillow. His blood pressure

has been in the range 150/90–150/100 mm Hg and his jugular venous pressure is at the normal level. John has never smoked.

Eating and drinking
After his heart attack 2 years ago, John was advised to stop adding salt to his food. He states that he enjoys food, and his usual eating pattern is a full cooked breakfast, a light lunch, and dinner with meat and plenty of vegetables. His weight has always been steady at 65 kg. He is not overweight.

Sleeping
John usually sleeps for 7–8 hours a night.

Mobilising
John has always been a very active person and has only recently curbed his activities because of chest pain and shortness of breath.

Communicating
John is very lively and animated and appears to be frank and open in conversation. He has a very positive self-concept and high self-esteem.

Perception of health state
John is curious about why he should have coronary artery disease. He is aware of the widely publicised 'risk factors' and feels strongly that he does not conform to the 'risk profile'. Nevertheless, John has accepted the diagnosis and the decision to operate. He is highly confident that he will return to his 'usual, if modified' lifestyle in about 3 months. He is a firm believer in homoeopathic remedies.

John's wife also seems to have accepted the situation. He thinks that she will 'cope' fairly well with his hospital stay and subsequent rehabilitation with help from the family.

Expressing sexuality
John has a very positive view of self. He and his wife have a satisfying sexual relationship. He can envisage no future problems.

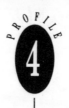

Working and playing

John has worked for a walking-stick manufacturer for 37 years and describes himself as a 'working manager'. His job has a high level of hard physical work, and he expresses concern about losing his heavy-goods-vehicle licence. In addition, John and his sons-in-law run their own business at weekends, laying drives and patios for other people. Work fills much of his time, and he has earned enough to have a very good lifestyle. John and his wife relax by going caravanning. He also does the gardening and enjoys listening to music.

Problems, expected outcomes, and interventions

This care study will not consider the period that John spent in the intensive care unit after surgery but will focus on the time that he spent in the general ward after transfer from intensive care, that is post-operative days 1–5.

Pre-operative preparation for John included shaving and application of skin disinfection, antibiotic prophylaxis, and a visit from the anaesthetist and intensive care unit nurse. The nurse explained about waking up in the unit, the presence of tubes, drains and lines, and some possible sensations that John would experience.

John spent less than 24 hours in the unit and has little memory of it. He was extubated fairly quickly on return, and the mediastinal and pericardial drains were removed before he returned to the ward.

Problem 1

Sleep deprivation. John states that he has not slept well since coming into hospital. He wakes about 2.00 am and then dozes on and off until the morning. He feels very tired for most of the day and has also had a disturbing nightmare.

Causes

Noise in the ward caused by staff activity and other patients; pain and discomfort related to operative incisions; anxiety related to post-operative progress.

Expected outcome

Sufficient quantity and quality of sleep to reduce perceived tiredness. He would like at least 6 hours uninterrupted.

Interventions

1. Give analgesia after 10.00 pm, as this allows John longer relief from discomfort after the lights have been turned out.
2. Ensure that he has the number of pillows which he likes.
3. Reduce noise in the ward to a minimum.
4. Allow time for sleep periods during the day.

PROFILE 4

Problem 2

Sternal wound pain and discomfort.

Causes
Sternotomy wounds produce high levels of muscular aches, pain and discomfort, while lack of sleep increases sensitivity to pain (McCauley and Polomano, 1980).

Expected outcomes
1. That the patient says that the pain and discomfort are controlled.
2. That the nurse will see that the patient is comfortable and able to contribute to his own recovery by moving about with ease; by deep breathing and coughing regularly, by interacting with his family in a relaxed manner and by active participation in daily hygiene and grooming activities.

Interventions
1. Assessment of pain can be carried out using the following guide:
   a. Consider the type of surgical pro-cedure, the presence of post-operative complications and the time that has elapsed since surgery.
   b. Evaluate the patient's perception of pain. This can be done by confirming whether or not he has pain and finding out where it is and its level— is it deep or is it superficial?
   c. Question the quality of the pain: sharp, piercing, dull, aching.
   d. Question the quantity of pain: mild, moderate, severe (or use a scale).
   e. Explore influencing factors: what makes it better; what makes it worse.
2. Evaluate the effect of analgesia.
3. Arrange for activities such as chest physiotherapy to be covered by analgesia.

Question 1

On a separate sheet of paper, list two more interventions which would help to reduce pain.

Problem 3

Potential post-operative wound infection.

Cause
Contamination of wounds by micro-organisms from various possible sources: patient's own flora; by cross-infection in the ward.

Expected outcome
Sternal wound
Healed and free from discomfort by 6–12 weeks.

Leg wounds
Dry and healed in 10–14 days.

Question 2

On a separate sheet of paper, list the interventions that would prevent this potential problem.

Question 3

On a separate sheet of paper, suggest any other problems which John might have. Make a list of their causes, expected outcomes, and interventions.

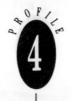

PROFILE

4

Rationale

After cardiac surgery, the patient has various actual and potential problems associated with both his activities of living and his lifestyle, and with alterations in physiology, particularly of the respiratory, cardiovascular and neurological systems. (For a full discussion of the immediate post-operative management see Shuldham (1984) and Weiland and Walker (1986).)

John states that the lack of sleep was his most distressing problem. Inability to obtain sufficient sleep, a vital basic need, is a common complaint among hospital patients (Hilton, 1976). Frequent sleep interruptions reduce not only the quantity but also the quality of sleep. Studies of cardiac surgery patients show that the sleep that is lost is mainly rapid-eye-movement sleep, and this appears to contribute to reports of more irritability, fatigue and increased sensitivity to pain, to feelings of lethargy and depression, and to post-cardiotomy delirium (McCauley and Polomano, 1980; Farrimond, 1984).

All efforts should be made to ensure adequate rest and comfort. Lengthy visiting periods with many relatives and friends can be very tiring.

Although pain control was not a major problem for John, it is not unusual for it to be so. In a follow-up study of post-operative coronary artery bypass graft (CABG) patients, Wilson-Barnett (1981) reports that about one-third of patients complained of sternal pain, and one-quarter complained of leg pain and swelling 1 year after surgery.

Proper relief of pain is one of the most important challenges to nurses. Inadequate pain relief can delay recovery.

The results of two recent British studies of post-operative wound infection in CABG patients report quite high rates of infection in both sternal and leg wounds. Wells *et al.* (1983) report a 12% infection rate (7.5% involving the sternal wound), and Farrington *et al.* (1985) found that sternal wounds were infected at the rate of 8.7% and leg wounds 12.9%.

Most researchers have found that wounds are infected by the patient's own skin flora, usually from the leg and groin, and are acquired in theatre. Prolonged hospital stay before surgery is known to promote infection, and this may be pertinent to this group of patients who regularly wait in hospital for space on an operating list. If transfer of organisms from legs to the chest occurs during surgery, then scrupulous pre-operative disinfection of the legs and groins is important (Cruse and Foord, 1980).

Showering or bathing with the use of skin disinfection has been shown to reduce post-operative infection and can be reduced further if it is done repeatedly (Brandberg *et al.*, 1980). This may be an indication for showers to be started before admission.

A reduction in wound infection in clean wounds can also be achieved by replacing razor shaves with chemical depilation, or doing the shave 2 hours before surgery (Cruse and Foord, 1980; *The Lancet*, 1983).

Rehabilitation should start pre-operatively and continue after discharge. Nurses have a key role in the teaching of patients before discharge and in running activity programmes and support groups.

Patients are still reporting lack of specific information and advice before discharge. Referring again to the study by Wilson-Barnett (1981), patients would certainly like guidance for activity graduation when home, perhaps in written form. This may serve to overcome the overprotectiveness of spouses reported by many patients (Stanton *et al.*, 1984).

Advice is also required on smoking, diet, weight, resumption of sexual activity, and driving. In addition, it is important that the patient knows the operation can be expected to contribute to a pain-free active life (Wilson-Barnett, 1981).

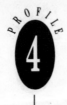
Evaluation

Problem 1

Sleep deprivation.

This problem was unresolved by day 5, despite analgesia timing to ensure a comfortable night. Noise, an uncomfortable bed and chest discomfort after 4 hours were still problematic. Analgesia was given again in the night but sleep was fitful. However, by this time John was due to be transferred back to his local hospital and hoped that lack of sleep would be less of a problem there.

Problem 2

Sternal wound pain.

John's perception of pain after the first 2 days was that the sternal pain was dull and aching and the leg wounds 'pulled'. Narcotic analgesia was needed for the first 2 days. After this, a milder oral analgesic every 4 hours was effective in keeping John comfortable. John was carrying out regular deep breathing and coughing. Auscultation and chest x-ray revealed no congestion or consolidation. He is increasing his activity level day by day and carrying out his own hygiene and grooming.

Problem 3

Potential wound infection.

Sternal wound
The appearance of the wound, and the presence of redness, swelling, localised pain and tenderness can be considered in evaluating the presence of infection. Temperature elevation should also be considered. It should be remembered that sternal pain can continue for many months.

Leg wounds
These have a tendency to ooze serous fluid, and delayed wound healing and swelling of the legs have been found to be a problem with a significant number of patients.

Answers to questions 1, 2 and 3

Problem 2

Question 1

Further interventions to reduce pain are:

1. Ensure that patient uses splinting technique for incision when coughing.

2. Provide an atmosphere which reinforces the patient's behaviour to seek pain relief.

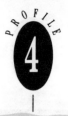
Problem 3

Question 2

Interventions to prevent wound infection are:

1. Pre-operatively, at least two showers or bath with application of skin disinfectant. If patient is being shaved, it should be done 2 hours or less before the operation or by chemical depilatory.
2. Remove dressing and spray sternal wound with plastic dressing on third or fourth day.
3. Dress leg wounds as necessary, and apply elastic stockings to alleviate the oedema. Elevate legs when sitting. Walk regularly.
4. Monitor for pyrexia.

Question 3

Another problem that John might have is anxiety related to recovery and future lifestyle.

Cause
1. Experience of angina and shortness of breath before surgery may adversely affect John's perceptions of future activity levels.
2. Concern regarding return to work.
3. Concern regarding the 'length of life of the grafts'.

Expected outcome
That John will be able to understand the reasons for surgery, and his possible health state in the future.

Intervention
Provide teaching sessions for John and his wife, which will meet the expected outcome.

Evaluation
John's level of knowledge can be evaluated during conversations, and any misconceptions can then be corrected.

A further problem might be weakness and fatigue in hospital and following discharge.

Cause
Related to having major cardiac surgery.

Expected outcome
1. Statements by John and his wife which show that they understand that this is a usual problem after surgery.
2. Gradual regaining of stamina.
3. Return to work by 3 months.

Intervention
Provide teaching sessions for John and Jean which outline the activity programme. Also provide guidelines which specify amount and intensity of exercise, and include those activities which should be avoided.

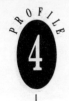

References

Brandberg, A., Holm, J., Hammersten, J., and Schersten, T. (1980). Post-operative wound infections in vascular surgery— effect of pre-operative whole body disinfection by shower-bath with chlorhexidine soap. *Royal Society of Medicine International Congress and Symposium Series*, No. 23, *Problems in the Control of Hospital Infection*, Royal Society of Medicine, London, pp. 71–75.

Cruse, P. J. E., and Foord, R. (1980). The epidemiology of wound infection. A 10-year prospective study of 62939 wounds. *Surgical Clinics of North America*, **1** (60), 27–40.

Farrimond, P. (1984). Post-cardiotomy delirium. *Nursing Times*, **80** (30), 39–41.

Farrington, M., Webster, M., Fenn, A., and Phillips, I. (1985). Study of cardiothoracic wound infection at St Thomas' Hospital. *British Journal of Surgery*, **72** (9), 759–762.

Hilton, B. A. (1976). Quantity and quality of patient's sleep and sleep disturbing factors in a respiratory intensive care unit. *Journal of Advanced Nursing*, **1**, 453–468.

McCauley, K., and Polomano, R. C. (1980). Acute pain: a nursing perspective with cardiac surgical patients. *Topics in Clinical Nursing*, **2** (1), 45–56.

Shuldham, C. (1984). Coronary artery surgery. *Nursing, Second Series*, **2** (25), 748–752.

Stanton, B., Jenkins, D., Savageau, J. A., Harken, D. L., and Aucoin, R. (1984). Perceived adequacy of patient education and fears and adjustments after cardiac surgery. *Heart and Lung*, **13** (5), 525–530.

The Lancet (1983). Pre-operative depilation (editorial). *The Lancet*, **i**, 1311.

Weiland, A. P., and Walker, W. E. (1986). Physiologic principles and clinical sequelae of cardiopulmonary bypass. *Heart and Lung*, **15** (1), 34–39.

Wells, F. C. M., Newson, S. W. B., and Rowlands, C. (1983). Wound infection in cardiothoracic surgery. *The Lancet*, **1**, 1209–1210.

Wilson-Barnett, J. (1981). Assessment of recovery: with special reference to a study with post-operative cardiac patients. *Journal of Advanced Nursing*, **6** (6), 435–445.

PROFILE

5

Lynn Batehup

An elderly lady who keeps falling:

Planning for safe mobility

Planning care is a practical exercise which must be adapted for individual patients. Some background information is provided about 84-year-old Mrs Barker who kept falling at home and who became incontinent. Following this, two nursing problems are outlined, together with their causes, expected outcomes and interventions. Identification of other reasons for Mrs Barker's problems is required and the expected outcomes and interventions need to be provided; the answers appear at the end of the chapter.

Patient profile

Mrs Elizabeth Barker is 84 years old and was admitted to hospital after several falls at home. This last fall had resulted in a fracture of the radius of the left arm. Her first admission, 8 weeks ago, had followed a fall injuring the right radius. Since discharge after the first fracture, Mrs Barker had fallen at home four times, during a period of about 2 weeks.

Assessment information
Biographical and social information
Mrs Barker is a widow—her husband had died 3 weeks before her first admission for right wrist fracture. She now lives alone in a first-floor flat in a fairly modern block. Her husband died following a perforated ulcer, aged 85. They had been married for 60 years. They had one son, who had died 2 years ago with cancer. Mrs Barker's daughter-in-law and grand-daughter live away and visit fairly infrequently.

Current health status
According to Mrs Barker, she has not had any major illnesses and has never been in hospital until the first admission 8 weeks ago. She sees herself as quite robust and healthy in general: 'I feel well in myself.' She does not know why she has started to fall. Table 5.1 shows the history of her two main falls.

Assessment
Safety in the environment
Mrs Barker has a compact flat consisting of a sitting room, bedroom, bathroom and kitchen. There is not much furniture to clutter the place. There are no loose rugs, floor lamps or trailing wires. Mrs Barker does not have to do any cooking except to make a cup of tea, for which she uses an electric kettle. She has had no accidents in the kitchen. A low armchair in her flat has been replaced by a higher upright one.

Table 5.1 History of two main falls

	First fall	Second fall
Time of day	Late afternoon	Mid-day
Place of fall	Sitting room	Sitting room
Activity before fall	Sitting in armchair	Eating lunch at small table
Activity during fall	Quiet walking	Quiet walking
Others present	No	No
Distractions during activity	Does not remember	Wanted to get the front door closed
Sensations experienced before fall such as dizziness, giddiness	None	None
Lighting	Daylight—bright	Daylight—bright
Floor covering	Fitted carpet	Fitted carpet
Obstacles	Cannot remember	Two armchairs
Time spent on floor following fall	About ½ hour	3 hours
Type of clothing and footwear	Husband's slippers Blouse and skirt	Own slippers Blouse and skirt
Sedative drugs	None	None

Eating and drinking
Mrs Barker has meals on wheels provided and she also has some help from neighbours.

Eliminating
Mrs Barker states that she is incontinent—she is aware of when she wants to micturate but cannot get to the lavatory in time. She has to get up several times at night but has never wet the bed. Thus, her incontinence pattern needs assessing. A urine specimen shows heavy growth of coliform bacilli. Since starting on antibiotics, Mrs Barker's incontinence has improved.

Communicating
Mrs Barker is very talkative and animated. She speaks in a clear lucid fashion. She has difficulty hearing a normal speaking tone in the right ear but there are no apparent difficulties on the left side. She needs glasses for reading. At present, she can read only large print in the newspaper and is due to have her eyes tested. This will be in hospital.

Working and playing
Mrs Barker has not worked outside the home for many years and had not been out of the flat since the falls started as she was frightened that she would fall in the street. She spends some time reading but needs new glasses—and watches some television. She does not feel lonely.

Sleeping
She has no problems in this area.

Personal cleansing
Mrs Barker manages her personal hygiene herself and has no problems.

Emotional state
Mrs Barker is still grieving over her husband's death: 'I feel numb; I am trying to get over it; I feel very depressed.' She never thought that she would be left alone—she had expected her son to look after her. When she sees other patients' visitors, she feels like crying, although outwardly she appears cheerful and likes to talk. She feels that she is resilient: 'I have managed to get through two world wars.'

Mobilising at home
When at home, Mrs Barker was able to walk around the flat. She was able to dress herself and to attend to her own hygiene. Although she was supposed to walk with a stick, she frequently did not.

Mobilising in the ward
In bed With her left arm in plaster and a sling, she is unable to rise from lying to sitting without help from another person.
Rising from a chair At the time of assessment, Mrs Barker was unable to rise without help from the left side. She pushes down with her right arm and her feet are placed close together.
Standing balance She is unsteady because her feet are placed too close together and her knees and hips are flexed. Thus, she tends to sway backwards from the midline and laterally to the left side. She makes some attempt to correct the displacement by straightening her head and neck. When standing, she reaches out for a person or object nearby. When she was at home, she says, there was nothing to hold on to in the sitting room that did not move.
Walking She has a small stepped gait with a narrow stride, lifting her feet off the ground only slightly. She uses a stick in her right hand but does not lean on it. She finds it difficult to move forwards without verbal and physical help from the left side. As she sways posteriorly, she needs constant reminders to stand up straight. It takes only a gentle push to the sternal area to cause a loss of balance laterally to the left or posteriorly.
Turning This is not done during forward movement. Anxiously, she takes small tottering steps and is easily off balanced.
Approaching chair She stops about 18 in from the chair and tends to lunge at it.
Sitting This is fairly controlled. Mrs Barker lowers herself with help from the left. She has no dizziness or giddiness when she is standing, turning or walking.

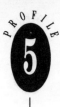

Blood pressure
No postural hypotension.

Pulse
90/min and regular.

24-hour electrocardiograph
Mostly sinus rhythm with runs of atrial fibrillation at up to 150/min. She was started on digoxin 125 μg once daily.

Problems, expected outcomes, and interventions

Problem 1

Repeated falls at home arising from uncorrected displacement of the body from its support base.

Cause 1
Impairment of postural control mechanisms, leading to decreased environmental perception, slowing of responses and weakness of support.

Figure 5.1 Components of the body's servomechanism which prevents falling

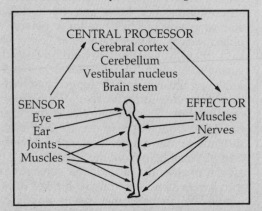

Expected outcomes
1. That Mrs Barker will be able to move around safely in a home environment that is free from hazards.
2. Will demonstrate safety in rising from sitting to standing.
3. Will demonstrate control over walking and turning.

4. Will demonstrate self-confidence in her ability to be mobile.

Interventions
A team approach will be used, involving the occupational therapist and physiotherapist who will assess the lay-out of the home for possible hazards.
A retraining programme for safe mobility at home will involve:

1. Wearing suitable clothes and shoes.
2. Eye test and hearing test.
3. Instilling a need for care and concentration when undertaking any activity.
4. Educating her to avoid sudden head and neck movements or looking upwards by hyperextending the neck, but learning to step carefully backwards instead.

Instruction and practice will be given in:

1. Rising from lying to sitting.
2. Rising from sitting to standing.
3. Standing to sitting.
4. Gaining standing balance.
5. Walking and turning.
6. Correct use of walking stick, at the same time assessing whether there is a need for other walking aids.
7. How to get up from the floor.

Cause 2
Transient circulatory impairment related to short episodes of atrial fibrillation.

Expected outcome
That Mrs Barker will have some understanding of her problem and therefore be able to state what medication she is taking, the dose, the time that she took it and any side-effects from it.

Interventions
Monitor apex and radial pulses for a limited period to assess the effects of her medication.

Provide short repetitive teaching sessions and evaluate.

Question 1

Now try to record on a separate sheet of paper at least two other possible causes of loss of postural control in this patient, with their expected outcomes and interventions.

Problem 2

Episodes of urinary incontinence. Aware of the need to micturate but cannot get to the lavatory in time. However, she does not wet the bed.

Cause
Mobility problems make it difficult to get to the lavatory on time. Perhaps she has a urinary tract infection.

Question 2

Although impaired mobility is making it difficult for Mrs Barker to get to the lavatory on time, there are other possible factors which may be relevant to this problem. On a separate sheet of paper, list some of these factors and the expected outcome and intervention for this patient.

Rationale

Recent studies of falls in old people at home have indicated that they are usually owing to a combination of extrinsic factors, such as poor lighting, slipping on rugs and other environmental hazards, and intrinsic factors, such as visual impairment, muscle weakness, postural hypotension, vertebrobasilar ischaemia, cervical spondylosis and cardiac dysrhythmias (Wild *et al.*, 1981a). Difficulties arise in determining the 'cause' of the fall, because it is shown that patients seldom remember exactly what happened, doctors and nurses rarely witness the fall, and physical signs are an indifferent guide to the transient disturbances of functions which provoke a fall (Wild *et al.*, 1981b).

Wild *et al.* (1981a) found little evidence that falls in old age are often caused by vertebro-

basilar ischaemia, cervical spondylosis and the like. It seems more common for falls in the elderly to result from errors in environmental perception, slowing of responses, and weakness of support. This is in line with the idea that falls result from uncorrected displacement of the body from its support base.

During everyday activities of standing, walking, stooping and so on, the body is constantly adjusting and maintaining the correct posture. Falls are prevented by the action of a servomechanism which has three components (Isaacs, 1978): the 'sensor' composed of visual, vestibular and proprioceptive elements; the 'central processor', consisting of brain areas such as brain stem, cerebellum, basal ganglia, sensorimotor cortex, etc; the 'effector' outflow from brain to spinal cord and peripheral nerves and muscles (Figure 5.1).

Studies of old people who fall have fou that certain elements of the balance mecha ism are impaired. These include 'postural sway' which is increased in people who fall because of loss of balance (Overstall *et al.*, 1977), poor vision (Campbell *et al.*, 1981), vestibular and vibration sense (Brocklehurst *et al.*, 1982), or slowing of maximal nerve conduction velocities especially in the lower limbs (Behse and Buchtal, 1971).

The gait of patients hospitalised after falling at home was shown to differ from others who had no history of falls. It is characterised by a slow speed, short step length, narrow stride width, wide range of stepping frequency, and large variability of step length (Guimaraes and Isaacs, 1980). The term 'post-fall syndrome' was coined by Murphy and Isaacs (1982) for the behaviour of some elderly patients following a fall. These patients expressed a great fear of falling when stood erect, tending to grab and clutch at objects within their view, and showing remarkable hesitancy and irregularity in their walking attempts. It seems that the post-fall syndrome was not present in the patients before they fell, but that it is the end point of a positive feedback spiral in which impaired balance leads to falls with further impaired balance.

Those at risk of falling are people aged 75 years and over who are house bound, who have an abnormal gait or a fear of falling and who walk with short irregular steps. Any

policy for the prevention of falls should put emphasis on the physical state of the faller. Hypnotics, sedatives and tranquillisers should not be prescribed for the very frail elderly person (Wild *et al.*, 1981a). It is important to record carefully the history of the falls. Information about events at the time of the fall may identify the cause of postural displacement, which may in turn lead to a guide for fall prevention.

When the patient is incontinent but aware of the need to micturate, attention to environmental factors can help to re-establish and maintain continence (KEHFL, 1983). It is important to assess the pattern of micturition. This is based on 2-hourly observation for a full 24 hours to discover whether the patient is wet or dry, and this is then recorded on a chart (Clay, 1980). the patient is then asked to pass urine and the result is recorded. If lavatory facilities are refused, this is also recorded. If, at the end of 2 hours, the patient is found to be incontinent, the time period can be shortened and, if the lavatory facilities are not needed so frequently, the interval can be lengthened.

Using this method, a pattern of micturition will become evident. This may take 1–2 weeks to emerge.

Using this information, patients with a defined pattern of micturition can now be considered for habit retraining.

The aim of this is to produce a socially acceptable lavatory rhythm by retraining the bladder from the starting point of the pattern shown (Wild *et al.*, 1981a).

Evaluation

Evaluation for this problem occurs over a lengthy period of retraining, and it is probably necessary to evaluate at weekly or fortnightly periods. Table 5.2 presents the activities and criteria for evaluation of the standing and walking re-education problem. At the same time a rationale for the action is given.

Mrs Barker's pattern of micturition showed that she was incontinent mainly in the late afternoon and early evening when there were few staff on duty. She therefore had to wait for lengthy periods before being helped to the lavatory. Her fluid intake was satisfactory and she was not constipated. There was no significant growth on her urine cul-

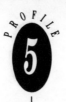

ture. So, for 2 weeks, a commode was placed by the bedside in the late afternoon and Mrs Barker was helped on to it. As her mobility improved, and she was able to walk short distances unaided, the periods of incontinence were reduced and after 4 weeks she stopped being incontinent.

Table 5.2 Post-fall walking retraining

Sitting to Standing	Rationale
Level of anxiety should be as low as possible: 1. Use arms to push down on arms of chair. 2. Flex knees, draw feet under the front edge of seat. 3. Bend trunk forward over thighs. 4. Rise by extending knees/hips, and straightening the trunk.	1. Downward push required for support and bracing of back muscles. Avoid using higher objects such as nearby tables, chairs or people, for pulling up on. 2. Feet placed close to front edge of chair. Feet placed apart to bring centre of gravity of the body over a wide base. 3. Bring body weight forwards far enough so that: 4. Weight is evenly distributed on the whole of the feet. If not, then weight taken on heels; hips remain flexed, causing a tendency to fall backwards on to the chair.
Standing to sitting 5. Bend trunk forward slightly. 6. Use arms to support and steady. 7. Flex hips and knees to sit. Straighten the trunk and sit back in the chair.	5. Leading with the head. 6. Putting one hand on the arm of the chair helps identify the position of the chair, and provides stability. 7. Should be performed in a controlled fashion.
Standing 1. Head and trunk should be erect. Hips and knees extended. Feet flat on the floor, slightly apart. Balance unsupported, or with usual aid.	1. A common problem is failing to complete extension, landing with flexed hips/knees. Postural sway is increased in elderly persons. Anteroposterior sway is affected mainly by articular, muscular and neurologic disorders. Lateral sway reflects mainly vestibular and visual defects.
Walking Provide calm support. If instructions are required, make clear, short, precise statements. Ensure patient understands what activity is to be carried out. 1. *Stance phase of walking—from standing* Body weight moved forward over the forward foot, with toes of near foot remaining on the ground to help maintain balance. 2. *Swing and heel strike* With support still on forward leg, the rear leg is lifted and flexed to clear the floor as it swings forward; the knee is extended and the foot dorsiflexed to allow the heel to be put on the ground—heel strike. This foot is now the supporting leg. The balanced support of the other leg must not be disturbed during practice of the swing and heel strike.	The ability to relax is important for anxious, elderly people who have lost their confidence owing to repeated falls. Muscular tension is reduced, and the patient tires less easily.

PROFILE 5

Table 5.2 (continued)

3. *Weight transference and return to stance*
Return to stance position occurs with the other foot forward. Body weight is then transferred from the rear leg to be supported over the forward leg.

Phases 2 and 3 are repeated alternately so the patient moves from one stance to the other. It should be practised until the move is a rhythmical walking pattern.

Elderly persons who have fallen tend to have an abnormal gait pattern:

1. Walking speed is slow.
2. Step length is short.
3. Step lengths are uneven—great variability.
4. Stride is narrow.

Walking is dominated by a desire to limit displacement beyond the support back to the minimum which the patient can handle and is accompanied by much anxiety.

Treatment aims to help the gait regain some normality and automaticity.

Answers to questions 1 and 2

Problem 1

Question 1

Other causes of loss of postural control might include:

Cause (a)
Loss of confidence and great anxiety—post-fall syndrome (Wild *et al.*, 1981a).

Expected outcome
An expressed feeling of confidence when undertaking activities, and that she shows she can move safely.

Intervention
As for Cause (a).

Cause (b)
Recent bereavement. Mrs Barker's husband had died three weeks before her first recorded fall. He had been a psychological and physical support for her.

Expected outcome
That she will express her present thoughts and feelings.

Intervention
Provide a supportive, caring atmosphere. Make time to listen and talk. Bereavement counselling is available; assess the need for it.

Problem 2

Question 2

Expected outcome
Re-establishment and maintenance of continence.

Intervention
1. Assess the pattern of micturition.
2. Place Mrs Barker nearer to the lavatory.
3. Assess her fluid intake.
4. Assess whether or not she is constipated.
5. Make sure the call bell and her stick or walking frame are near at hand.
6. Take a mid-stream specimen of urine for culture and sensitivity.

When the interventions have been carried out it should be possible to know whether habit retraining is appropriate. The questions that should be asked when trying to assess the factors that can help establish and maintain continence are:

1. What does the pattern of micturition show, and is the existing routine frequent enough for the patient's needs?
2. Are adequate toilet facilities—lavatory, commode or urinal—available and readily accessible? Relative heights of bed, chair and commode are important. Warmth and privacy are essential. Can clothing be managed quickly and easily?
3. If the patient is on diuretics, are they being given at the most suitable time? Are they still necessary?
4. Is there a reasonable fluid intake during the day? Is there a need to restrict drinks two or three hours before sleep?
5. Is night sedation impairing awareness of the need to micturate and so causing bed-wetting?
6. Is the patient constipated?
7. Are walking aids such as sticks and walking frames readily accessible for use?

References

Behse, F., and Buchtal, F. (1971). Normal sensory conduction in the nerves of the leg in man. *Journal of Neurology, Neurosurgery and Psychiatry*, **34**, 404.

Brocklehurst, J. C., Robertson, D., and James-Groom, P. (1982). Clinical correlates of sway in old age—sensory modalities. *Age and Aging*, **11**, 1–10.

Campbell, A. J., Reinken, J., and Martinez, G. S. (1981). Falls in old age: a study of frequency and related clinical factors: *Age and Aging*, **10**, 264–270.

Clay, E. (1980). Rehabilitative nursing. In: Mandelstam, D. (ed.), *Incontinence and its Management*, Croom Helm, London.

Guimaraes, R. M., and Isaacs, B. (1980). Characteristics of the gait in old people who fall. *International Rehabilitation Medicine*, **2**, 177–180.

Isaacs, B. (1978). Are falls a manifestation of brain failure? *Age and Aging*, **7**, suppl., 97–105.

KEHFL (1983). *Action on Incontinence*, King Edward's Hospital Fund for London, London.

Murphy, J., and Isaacs, B. (1982). The post-fall syndrome. *Gerontology*, **28**, 265–270.

Overstall, P. W., Exton-Smith, A. N., Imms, F. J., and Johnson, A. L. (1977). Falls in the elderly related to postural imbalance. *British Medical Journal*, **1** (6056), 261–264.

Wild, D., Nayak, U. S. L., and Isaacs, B. (1981a). Description, classification and prevention of falls in old people at home. *Rheumatology and Rehabilitation*, **20**, 153–159.

Wild, D., Nayak, U. S. L., and Isaacs, B. (1981b). How dangerous are falls in old people at home? *British Medical Journal*, **282**, 266–268.

Lynn Batehup

Symptom control for a patient with breast cancer:

Planning for comfort

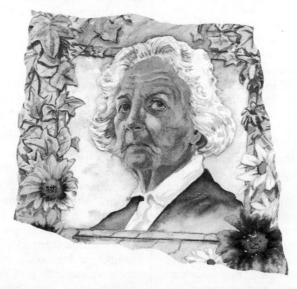

Emily Woods was admitted to hospital with pain from bone metastases after a mastectomy for breast cancer 10 years previously. She was also nauseated as a result of chemotherapy. Suggestions are made as to how these problems might be reduced. Also any further problems that Emily might have and the interventions you would make need to be considered; the answers are given at the end of the chapter.

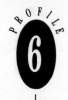

Patient profile

Emily Woods is a single woman aged 72 who lives with her younger sister in their own semidetached house in a London suburb. Emily describes the house as being 'convenient' for their use, with a large garden in which she spends as much time as possible. Emily's sister goes out to work daily from 8.30 am to 2.30 pm. Emily had been employed as a civil servant for all her working life until her retirement at the age of 63 because of ill health.

Assessment information
Previous health
Emily discovered a lump in her left breast in 1973 and, for a period of 3 years, she kept this information to herself because she was fearful of the consequences and thought it might go away on its on. In fact, she actively avoided routine medical examinations for this period of time, in an effort to keep it to herself. During this time, Emily experienced no symptoms apart from a 'pulling sensation' around the breast on the left side when she was lying in bed at night. In the event, the lump was discovered at a routine annual medical examination carried out by her employers, and the eventual outcome was that Emily had a mastectomy a short time later. Following the operation and convalescence, Emily returned to work and was seen by her doctor at regular intervals. Time between the check-ups decreased over the years and until 1983 were being carried out yearly. In 1983, Emily started to have pain in her right hip, and following examination by cancer specialists she was told that she had metastases in the bone. At present Emily is aware that she has bone metastases involving her ribs, pelvis and spine. Throughout the years, Emily has had endocrine therapy according to the progression of the disease.

Present health
In early 1985, Emily had pain from bone metastases in her right hip and ribs, and also had some tumour recurrence on her left chest wall, a mobile lump measuring 1 cm × 1 cm.

She was treated with endocrine therapy, and the lump got smaller and the pain was relieved. In April of this year, Emily was admitted to hospital for pain control related to bone secondaries. She received treatment with a three-drug combination of cytotoxic chemotherapy. The side-effects of vomiting and diarrhoea made it a 'terrible experience' for her.

In September, 1986 Emily was again admitted with pain and pathological fractures in her ribs. She was also found to have elevated levels of calcium in her blood. One dose of a three-drug combination of cytoxic drugs was given, and fluid replacement via the intravenous route was carried out.

Assessment
Communicating
Emily appears calm and collected. She responds to questions thoughtfully and carefully. She never at any time used the word cancer.

Perception of health state
Emily is well informed and aware of her condition. She knows that she has secondary deposits in the bone. She states that, when she first saw her operation scar, she was shocked and wanted 'to talk to someone who would understand'. Now, years later, she feels vulnerable and not in control of her own life and body. She also wishes that she had never taken full health for granted and often thinks 'Why me?' She states that she now lives a day at a time.

Eating and drinking
Emily's appetite is usually fairly good. A usual day would consist of tea and toast for breakfast, a snack for lunch, and a meal in the evening. Meals are provided by her sister. At present, her appetite is poor, and she has been feeling nauseated for the last 2 or 3 days. On admission, her serum calcium level was found to be elevated, 3.39×10^9/litre (normal range, 2.15–2.70×10^9/litre). A low-calcium diet was prescribed. Her mouth and

mucous membranes feel dry. There is no pain or signs of ulceration or stomatitis. Fluid intake is being increased by the administration of 3 litres of normal saline intravenously over 24 hours.

Elimination
Urinary   Usual pattern is to go two to three times a day. Experiences no problems. Ward test of urine showed no abnormalities.
Faecal   Usual pattern is once a day. Has recently been constipated over the last 3–4 days.

Breathing
Cardiovascular function is satisfactory. Emily sleeps lying on two pillows. Her blood pressure was 130/80 mmHg and her pulse 88 and regular. There is no visible oedema of the ankles, and jugular venous pressure is normal.

Mobilising
Within the past 6 weeks, Emily has started to use a wheelchair for getting around outside the house. Inside the house she can manage to get around using a stick. She is able to walk around the ward. The problem is related to pain in her right hip. Being jolted in the wheelchair over kerbs can also be a problem as too much of this causes pain at the sites of bone metastases. At present, pain relief is given by slow-release morphine sulphate tablets 20 mg twice a day, and indo-methacin suppositories twice a day. Emily describes the pain as sharp; it is located in the right side of her back, and on a scale of 0–10 its intensity is 5. It is only present on movement.

Sleep
Usually sleeps well, from 10.00 pm to 6.00 am. Is not sleeping well at present.

Work and play
Emily has worked as a civil servant until retirement at the age of 63. It was a responsible job where she was running a department of some 30 people. She enjoyed it and was reluctant to retire. Emily has always had an active social life. She goes on holiday abroad each year with a woman-friend and has been on many enjoyable cruises. At present, Emily is spending much of her time reading and, when the weather permits, lies in the sun in the garden.

Safety in the environment
Emily may be at risk of developing an infection because of impaired immune defences. On admission, her haemoglobin and white-cell count were within normal limits, her temperature is normal and all skin surfaces are clean and intact. Following chemotherapy, her haemoglobin is 9.2 g/dl (normal range, 13–18 g/dl), and her white cell count is 1.3×10^9/litre (normal range, $4–11 \times 10^9$/litre).

Problems, expected outcomes, and interventions

Problem 1

Loss of appetite and nausea for 3 days. Emily did not vomit but felt continuously nauseated, and unable to eat or drink.

Causes
1. Hypercalcaemia. Her serum calcium level is 3.39×10^9/litre.
2. Cytotoxic chemotherapy.

Expected outcomes
1. Patient's statement that nausea is relieved.
2. Adequate hydration for reduction of calcium levels.
3. Return of appetite and usual eating pattern.

Interventions
1. Give the anti-emetic drug prescribed. Check its effect 20 min after administration.
2. Monitor the intravenous infusion of normal saline 1 litre 8-hourly.

Question 1

What other interventions would be helpful in the relief of this problem?

Problem 2

Pain in right lower back, described as sharp, 'mainly occurs when I move', intensity reported as 5 on a scale 0–10.

Cause
Metastatic bone lesions secondary to cancer of the breast.

Expected outcomes
1. Patient's statement that the pain is absent or controlled to her expectations.
2. Comfortable movement and activity.

3. Maintenance of usual bowel pattern— absence of constipation.

Question 2

What interventions would help to relieve this problem?

Question 3

What other problems might be experienced by this patient?

Rationale

Breast cancer is now one of the chief causes of death for women in many countries of the world (*Manual of Clinical Oncology*, 1982). As with a large number of malignant tumours the cause of breast cancer is far from being well understood. Epidemiological studies as well as experimental and clinical research indicate that certain groups of women have a higher risk than others of developing cancer of the breast. Women with a family history of breast cancer appear to have an increased risk; parity also seems an important risk factor, with nulliparous women being more susceptible than those women who have had children; an early first pregnancy has been shown to confer protection on the woman, but lactation has not been proved a protecting factor (*Manual of Clinical Oncology*, 1982).

Breast cancer is regarded as a systemic and chronic disease as eventually most patients will develop local and distant metastases requiring various forms of endocrine and cytotoxic chemotherapy determined by the progression of the disease and sites involved (Smith, 1985). Breast cancer may spread locally, regionally to lymph nodes, and distantly to various sites in the body. In breast cancer the most frequent site for spread of distant metastases is in the bone, followed by the lung, liver and brain (Fisher *et al.*, 1977; *Manual of Clinical Oncology*, 1982).

Hypercalcaemia is a fairly common complication of breast cancer and is related to widespread skeletal metastases (Bondy, 1978). The process of increased bone resorption exceeds the kidney's capacity to excrete calcium, and so the serum calcium concentration rises. Dehydration may make the hypercalcaemia worse. When the hypercalcaemia is mild, it causes constipation and lethargy and, when more severe, it produces distressing symptoms such as nausea, vomiting, anorexia, weakness and mental dullness (*British Medical Journal*, 1984). Commonly, these symptoms may be attributed to the malignant condition or to the side-effects of chemotherapy or radiotherapy. The mainstay of treatment is by rehydration and forced saline diuresis with intravenous saline and diuretics to optimise and increase the renal excretion of calcium (*British Medical Journal*, 1984). Drugs are available for the treatment of this condition (for a review, see *British Medical Journal* (1984) and Selby *et al.* (1984)). It is necessary for the patient to be made aware of the possibility that this condition might arise, and what symptoms to look out for.

Bone metastases may not always be painful. Those that are cause pain in a variety of ways. These include local bone pain, radiation into surrounding tissues, referred pain, nerve compression, muscle spasm and associated myofascial pain (Twycross and Lack, 1983). Local bone pain ranges from a dull ache to a deep oppressive intense pain. With a pathological rib fracture the pain is most intense when changing from sitting to lying positions or vice versa. In many instances the patient expects that the nurse will know all about her pain, assuming the pain to be typical and needing no further explanation. Similarly, the nurse may rely on the patient's telling her about the pain (Raiman, 1981). These

unspoken assumptions may result in the patient's enduring unnecessary pain, whilst the nurse is under the impression that pain is controlled. This points to the need for a regular structured pain assessment and review of analgesia (Raiman, 1981). In addition, informing and explaining to the patient the cause of pain, and the details of the drugs used, is fundamental to successful pain control. The patient needs to understand in order to make sense of what is happening and to be able to participate effectively.

The most common cause of reduced white cell counts, and reduction in other blood cells in patients with non-haematological malignancies, is cytoxic chemotherapy and radiotherapy (Ristuccia, 1985). The ability of the patient's immune system to withstand infection is impaired. Nurses taking care of oncology patients need to have a sound knowledge of the disease pathology as well as an understanding of the effects of the therapy used to treat malignancy, considering the spectrum of side-effects encountered from chemotherapy. These drugs affect most major body systems as well as simultaneously attacking the patient's cancer. Chemotherapy interfers with the ability of the bone marrow to produce red cells, white cells and platelets. Nurses should be alert to signs of infection in these patients and protect them from obvious sources of infection such as other patients or family members.

For many people, illness in general and cancer in particular create a sense of helplessness. It seems to patients that their life is completely in the hands of others, most frequently the hands of doctors and nurses. For most people, and more specifically for strongly independent people, this can prove extremely difficult. If patients can assume as much responsibility for their own care as possible, it will make them feel less dependent and more productive. Helping patients to help themselves means that patients need to be informed about their disease and to be taught skills for the management of their treatment and its consequences.

Evaluation

Problem 1

Loss of appetite and nausea.

Emily found that the most effective anti-emetic for her was domperidone, a drug regularly used for prevention and relief of nausea and vomiting especially when associated with cytotoxic drug therapy. This was given regularly and gave rapid relief. Intravenous fluid was given at the rate of 3 litres/24 hours for a period of 4 days. There was no evidence of cardiopulmonary side effects. Calcium levels reached normal levels in 4 days. Low-calcium diet was prescribed.

Problem 2

Back pain.

Emily reduced the level of pain that she experienced with controlled-release morphine sulphate 20 mg every 12 hours. Described as 3 on the scale 0–10 and dull. The non-steroidal anti-inflammatory drug indomethacin was also given; in addition, palliative chemotherapy was given. The result was some discomfort in Emily's back which she felt that she could tolerate.

Answers to questions 1, 2 and 3

Problem 1

Question 1

Interventions
As well as Interventions 1 and 2 already given, the following would be helpful:

3. Give the patient ice chips or cubes to suck.
4. Maintain comfort and cleanliness in the mouth with mouthwashes and oral toilet.
5. Position in a relaxed upright position well supported with pillows.
6. Give support and comfort.
7. Teach the patient about the importance of maintaining a good fluid intake, and help her to achieve this whilst in hospital.

PROFILE

6

Problem 2

Question 2

Interventions

1. Assess the pain using patient's subjective report and pain scale (Bourbonnais, 1981).
2. Ensure that analgesia is given promptly and regularly at the times prescribed. Monitor its effects. Review as necessary.
3. Use short regular teaching sessions to inform the patient of her drug regime, effects and side-effects such as constipation related to morphine (Doyle, 1984).
4. Assess the need for a regular colonic stimulant once or twice a day.
5. Advise the patient regarding an adequate fluid intake.
6. Advise the patient regarding fibre-rich foods.
7 Give time for Emily to ventilate her thoughts and feelings in a warm supportive relationship.

Question 3

As well as Problems 1 and 2, the following problems can arise.

Problem 3

Potential risk of acquired infection related to leukopenia—white-cell count, 1.3×10^9/litre (normal range, $(4-11) \times 10^9$/litre).

Causes

1. Bone marrow depression related to cytotoxic chemotherapy given for symptom control and relief.
2. Neoplastic process.

Expected outcome

Absence of infection as indicated by apyrexia, usual pulse and blood pressure, clear chest and airway, absence of dysuria, and clean mouth, teeth and gums.

Interventions

1. Nurse in a single room during risk period until the white-cell count is higher than 4×10^9/litre.
2. Adhere to principles of asepsis including stringent handwashing behaviour.
3. Help patient to maintain high standards of personal hygiene including mouth and teeth.
4. Monitor temperature and other vital signs regularly.
5. Help the patient to have a nutritious and appetising diet.
6. Ensure deep breathing and coughing regularly.
7. Monitor for signs of mouth soreness, sore throat, cough, congestion and dysuria.

Evaluation

Emily required 3 pints of blood; this increased her haemoglobin level and white-cell count to 12.2 g/dl and 3.1×10^9/litre, respectively. Temperature remained at or below 37 °C. Throughout her stay, no evidence of infection was present.

PROFILE 6

Problem 4

Perceived loss of control over her lifestyle and body function.

Causes
1. Insufficient knowledge about treatment regime and effects.
2. Uncertainty, fears and anxieties about the future effects of the neoplastic condition.

Expected outcome
An informed participant in her own care, leading to a feeling of some control over her own life.

Interventions
1. Provide information and teaching for the patient about:
   a. Therapeutic interventions and investigations.

b. Control of symptoms.
c. Possible future outcomes.
2. Facilitate patient participation in decision-making process and own self-care activities.
3. Help the patient to identify her fears and worries by 'active listening' (Maguire, 1985) and development of a trusting relationship.

Evaluation
Emily expressed fears about further chemotherapy and following discussion between her and her doctor, when full explanations were given about future dosage and type of therapy, she made the decision to carry on with it. She received teaching about pain relief medication and took an active part in her own pain assessment.

References

Bondy, P. K. (1978). Systemic manifestations of malignant tumours. In Tiffany, R. (ed.), *Oncology for Nurses and Health Care Professionals*, Vol. 1, George Allen and Unwin, London.

Bourbonnais, F. (1981). Pain assessment: development of a tool for the nurse and the patient. *Journal of Advanced Nursing*, **6**, 277–282.

British Medical Journal (1984). Treatment of hypercalcaemia associated with malignancy (editorial). *British Medical Journal*, **288**, 812–813.

Doyle, D. (1984). Pain control in terminal disease. *Cancer Care*, **1** (4), 8–10.

Fisher, B., Montague, E., Redmond, C. *et al*. (1977). Comparison of radical mastectomy with alternative treatments for a primary breast cancer. *Cancer*, **39**, 2827–2839.

Maguire, P. (1985). Towards more effective psychological interventions in patients with cancer. *Cancer Care*, **2** (2), 12–15.

Manual of Clinical Oncology (1982), 3rd edn, Springer, Berlin.

Raiman, J. (1981). Responding to pain. *Nursing, First Series*, **31**, 1362–1365.

Ristuccia, A. M. (1985). Haematologic effects of cancer chemotherapy. *Nursing Clinics of North America*, **20** (1), 235–239.

Selby, P. C., Peacock, D. H. and Marshall, D. H. (1984). Hypercalcaemia Management. *British Journal of Hospital Medicine*, **31** (3) 186–197.

Smith, I. E. (1985). Controversies in the medical management of breast cancer. *Postgraduate Medical Journal*, **61**, 117–122.

Twycross, R. G. and Lack, S. A. (1983). *Symptom Control in Far Advanced Cancer: Pain Relief*, Pitman, London.

Sue Adams and Gary Tubman

Drug overdose:

Planning sensitive care in the accident and emergency department

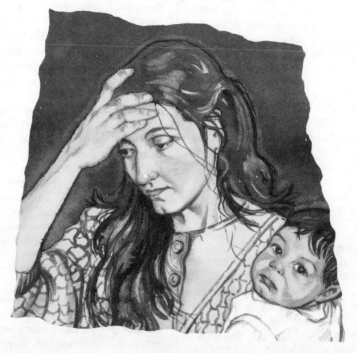

Jane had taken an overdose of para-
cetamol after becoming depressed at not being able to cope at
home. Some of the problems associated with overdose patients
are outlined. Description of the expected outcomes and interventions for these are required, together with suggestions on
how to assist Jane's family to accept what has happened in
order to give her the support that she needs; the answers are
at the end of the chapter.

Patient profile

Jane is 20 years old and was admitted to the accident and emergency (A&E) department on Thursday evening at 9.30 pm, having taken an overdose of approximately 25 paracetamol tablets with gin. She telephoned her aunt as soon as she had done this to ask her to look after her baby. On arriving at Jane's flat some 10 min later, her aunt telephoned for an ambulance and informed Jane's parents, who came to the A&E department. Her aunt stayed with the baby and said that she would leave a message for Jane's boy-friend when he returned home.

Assessment information
Biographical and social information
Jane lives with her boy-friend in a seventh-floor two-bedroom council flat in a large estate in South London. They have lived together for nearly 2 years and have a 9-month-old baby girl. Jane's parents live nearby and she sees them about once a week, and she has an aunt with whom she is very close.

Current health status
Jane was admitted to the A&E department conscious but a little drowsy. She responded to verbal commands and was able to move herself from the ambulance trolley to the casualty trolley. She was sitting upright. Her blood pressure was 105/65 mmHg, pulse 92 and respiration rate was 16/min. Her pupils were equal and reacting to light. Her breath smelt of alcohol. There were no signs that she had vomited. Jane's parents arrived shortly after the ambulance. Her father expressed annoyance about his daughter's actions. Her boy-friend did not arrive in casualty while she was there.

Assessment
Communication
Initially, Jane was very withdrawn, avoided eye contact and would not speak. This represented the first problem on her arrival in the A&E department.

Working and playing
Jane is untrained and unemployed. Her boy-friend works as a labourer. Jane usually goes out to the pub with her aunt about once a week. Her boy-friend, however, is out most evenings and usually returns late at night in a drunken and abusive state.

Emotional state
By speaking to her in a sympathetic manner, Jane began to confide that she felt very down and depressed and that she was no longer able to cope with the situation at home. She said that the baby was very tiring and cried a lot. She also said she was beginning to dread her boy-friend getting in at night. He is fairly rough with her although he has not beaten her up, and she does not think that he would harm the baby. She is able to confide in her aunt but has spoken very little to her parents about the problems.

Following the medical procedures in the A&E department, and shortly before being taken to the medical ward, Jane expressed her anxiety at the involvement of the social services and whether this would mean that her child would be taken into care.

Sleeping
Jane said that she has not been sleeping well over the past 2 or 3 weeks. She says she cannot get to sleep until her boy-friend has returned and settled down for the night, which is some time after midnight, and she is awoken by the baby at about 6.00 am.

Physical appearance
Jane is an attractive slim young woman, dressed in a T-shirt and jeans. She was not dirty or unkempt.

Assessment by therapist
The assessment of Jane took place on the medical ward the morning after she had taken the overdose by a psychiatric charge nurse.

Initially, Jane felt very embarrassed by the overdose and at being treated in hospital. Despite feeling nervous during the interview,

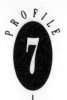

Jane gave a good account of herself and her present situation which she described as 'intolerable'.

She said that she did not want to die but felt helpless. She had not thought of taking an overdose prior to that night. On the evening of the overdose she was tired and felt 'cooped up' and that her baby girl 'would not stop crying'.

The therapist encouraged Jane to express her feelings of helplessness during the session and, although Jane was frequently tearful, she also felt relieved that she could talk to someone.

There was no evidence of psychiatric disorder, but it was clear that Jane was undergoing a considerable amount of stress and that paradoxically she had begun to seek help by taking the overdose.

Jane's aunt brought Jane's baby to visit her on the ward which eased her anxieties that the baby may be taken away because of the overdose. With Jane's permission, the therapist talked briefly with her aunt. Jane often confided in her and it was agreed that Jane could stay with her aunt when she was discharged from hospital later that evening.

The therapist discussed with Jane how she might be helped and what resources were available to her. It was arranged that the therapist would meet Jane the following day for an out-patient appointment to identify problems, and following that she would have four treatment sessions at weekly intervals.

Problems, expected outcomes, and interventions

Problems 1–3 are problems that require immediate attention, and Problems 4–9 are problems that can be dealt with when Jane returns for her four sessions at weekly intervals. Problems 1–3 were identified in the A&E department and the remainder when the patient was on the ward a day later.

Problem 1

Jane is uncommunicative and avoids eye contact with the nurse.

Cause
Presumed serious emotional problem as she has taken an overdose.

Expected outcome
That Jane will feel able to discuss her reasons for taking the overdose and her intentions.

Interventions
1. Give Jane the maximum opportunity to talk in private.
2. Show interest, concern and a desire to help.

Problem 2

The potential problem that Jane will develop severe hepatic impairment, possibly resulting in death.

Cause
Ingestion of 25 paracetamol (12.5 g), which is hepatotoxic, 45 min before her arrival in the A&E department.

Expected outcome
That Jane will not be at risk of hepatic failure and will co-operate with the stomach wash-out procedure.

Interventions
1. Gain Jane's co-operation by explaining the need for a stomach wash-out and exactly what this entails.
2. Wash out her stomach.
3. Administer methionine (paracetamol antidote) orally, 2.5 g every 4 hours up to 10 g total.
4. Take blood sample 4 hours after ingestion for paracetamol levels.

Question 1

On a separate piece of paper, list three risks associated with a stomach wash-out and how these can be avoided.

Problem 3

Potential respiratory depression.

Cause
The drinking of an unknown amount of alcohol.

Question 2

On a separate piece of paper, describe the expected outcome and the interventions to reduce the risk of respiratory depression.

Question 3

On a separate piece of paper, describe one further problem that requires immediate attention concerning Jane's family.

Problem 4

Poor relationship between Jane and her boy-friend.

Cause
Probably multiple, but boy-friend often threatening and abusive.

Expected outcome
Jane will be provided with the opportunity to look at how she will resolve the conflicts between them.

Interventions
1. Provide a safe comfortable environment conducive to talking.
2. Employ counselling skills.
3. Provide structure to the session.

Problem 5

Feelings of helplessness.

Cause
Jane feels that she is unable to cope with her 9-month-old baby daughter. Feeling helpless causes low self-esteem.

Expected outcome
She will feel able to help herself and cope with her baby.

Interventions
1. As in Problem 4.
2. As in Problem 4.
3. As in Problem 4.

Question 4

What additional interventions would help to relieve this problem?

Problem 6

Social isolation.

Cause
Jane lives in a seventh-floor flat. She is unemployed and has no hobbies and only an aunt to whom she is close.

Expected outcome
She will feel able to contact old friends, associations such as those for single-parent families, toddler groups and self-help groups.

Interventions
1. As in Problem 4.
2. As in Problem 4.
3. As in Problem 4.
4. Help her to look at her life and relationships prior to her having a baby and in the present situation.
5. Suggest re-establishment of contact.

Problem 7

Unsuitable accommodation.

Cause
Jane shares a small seventh-floor flat with her boy-friend on a large housing estate.

Expected outcome
Jane will look at her accommodation.

Interventions
1. As in Problem 4.
2. As in Problem 4.
3. As in Problem 4.
4. Refer to a social worker with Jane's consent.

Problem 8

Anxiety about social service involvement.

Cause
Jane feels that the social services may take her child away as she has taken an overdose.

Expected outcome
Jane will feel able to approach and trust the community services, such as the social worker and health visitor.

Interventions
1. As in Problem 4.
2. As in Problem 4.
3. As in Problem 4.
4. Explore why she feels this way.
5. Reassure, explaining the reality of community service involvement and their positive supporting role.

Problem 9

Reluctance to ask for emotional support from her parents.

Cause
Jane feels unable to talk to her parents regarding her problems.

Expected outcome
She will feel able to approach her parents and ask them 'What stops us talking to each other?'

Interventions
1. As in Problem 4.
2. As in Problem 4.
3. As in Problem 4.
4. Explore Jane's feelings.
5. Provide an environment and help Jane and her parents to enter into a dialogue with each other.

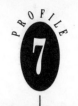

Rationale

Deliberate drug overdose is a common problem in A&E departments. It has been estimated that 110 000 cases of overdose present each year, with 82% of these being admitted and accounting for 14% of all medical admissions (Walsh, 1982).

The majority of patients who attempt suicide (parasuicide) have no intention of killing themselves. In a study of 216 parasuicides, Stanley (1969) found that less than one-quarter had a suicidal intent. Kreitman (1977) describes parasuicide as being carried out at the height of interpersonal crisis, an act which is used as a form of communication and which is designed to give relief from intolerable distress. Studies have shown that alcohol has been taken by 25% of parasuicides (Morgan *et al.*, 1975; Hawton and Catalan, 1987).

Overdosing is approximately five times more frequent in inner urban and council housing areas than in rural areas (Walsh, 1982), and between 1.5 and 2.1 times more women attempt suicide than do men (Hawton and Catalan, 1987).

Paracetamol is one of the drugs used in 40% of parasuicides (Hawton and Catalan, 1987) because of the ease with which it can be obtained. However, it is one of the most toxic drugs with as few as 20 tablets (10 g) causing hepatotoxicity and possible death; 96% of paracetamol is metabolised into non-toxic byproduct and excreted unchanged, but 4% is metabolised into a highly toxic substance. At therapeutic levels, this is rendered harmless by reacting with a naturally occurring substance, glutathione (Macy, 1979), but in overdose there is insufficient glutathione available and the free toxic metabolite bonds to hepatic cells, causing liver necrosis (Michell *et al.*, 1974). Symptoms of hepatotoxicity begin to occur after 24 hours and, after 48 hours, jaundice, coagulation defects, hypoglycaemia, renal failure and myocardiopathy may become obvious (Rumack and Matthews, 1975). Early emergency treatment is indicated.

A stomach wash-out is recommended for overdoses of 20 tablets or more if ingested within 6 hours (Cosgriff and Anderson, 1984). Antidotes are effective if given within the 24 hours after ingestion and bind with the toxic metabolite. Either methionine given orally or Parvolex (*N*-acetylcysteine) intravenously are used. Blood samples are taken 4 hours after ingestion to assess the risk of hepatotoxicity (Figure 7.1). Charcoal should not be given post-stomach wash-out if paracetamol is involved as it binds to the oral antidote (Cosgriff and Anderson, 1984).

The stomach wash-out also serves to remove the alcohol, although this generally would not be indicated if it were the only drug involved. Alcohol causes respiratory depression and in large quantities can cause respiratory arrest (Cosgriff and Anderson, 1984). The level at which this occurs varies

Figure 7.1 The Rumack–Matthews nomogram for paracetamol poisoning (Macy, 1979): a plot of paracetamol level against time

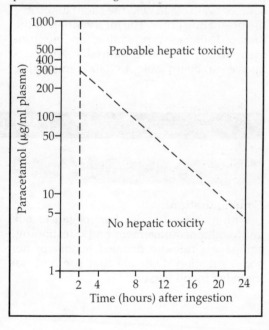

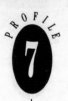

considerably between individuals, but 300–400 mg alcohol/100 ml blood can be potentially life threatening. Hypoglycaemia can result from excess alcohol intake as alcohol inhibits gluconeogenesis. This usually occurs 6–18 hours after ingestion.

The notion that stomach wash-out teaches the overdose patient a lesson is unsupported. Besides questioning the ethics of such a rationale, Walsh (1985), from a behaviourist theory viewpoint, doubts that parasuicides see the stomach wash-out as a punishment but rather see it in terms of receiving some of the help and attention which they need and desire.

The majority of parasuicides have no psychiatric illness (Stanley, 1969). The DHSS (1984) suggested a multidisciplinary approach to the care of such patients and that workers other than psychiatrists could assess patients. Brooking and Minghella (1987) reported on a study where community psychiatric nurses were considered the most appropriate therapist for parasuicides.

The initial assessment by the therapist aims to assess both the immediate and the future risks of suicide, the evidence of psychiatric illness, the current medical, social, psychological and financial problems, and the resources available to help the client to resolve the presenting crisis. The intervention of the therapist includes providing an environment which is safe, comfortable and conducive to being able to talk, employing counselling skills such as those described by Egan (1982) including being non-judgemental, empathic, genuine and respectful, and providing structure to the session.

Current literature suggests that a problem-solving approach is appropriate for counselling parasuicides (Hawton and Catalan, 1987). The approach needs to be flexible and tailored to individual needs. For Jane, the assessment by the therapist (in this case a psychiatric nurse) took place on the ward the morning following her overdose. It was arranged that she would be seen the following day as an out-patient where problems would be identified, and consequently treatment sessions would begin. The client is encouraged to take as much responsibility as possible for identifying problems, setting attainable goals and developing and utilising the necessary skills to achieve the goals.

Continued support in the community by both formal carers, such as the health visitor and social worker, and informal carers, such as self-help groups and family are instrumental in helping people such as Jane to cope in society. Babies whose mothers are young, immature, unsupported and under stress belong to one of the high-risk child abuse categories (Brandon, 1976).

Much care and time must be taken with parasuicides in order to determine their needs and to begin to help them to solve their problems. This is a challenging area to nursing.

Evaluation

Problem 1

Communication.

Within about 10 min, Jane began to talk and, with encouragement and questioning, she gave a full and detailed history of her social situation. She said that she had not intended to kill herself.

Problem 2

The risk of hepatotoxicity.

Jane agreed to have a stomach wash-out and coped well with the procedure. Tablet particles were retrieved.

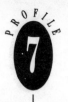

Problem 3

The risk of respiratory depression.
During her stay in the A&E department (approximately 2½ hours), Jane's level of consciousness remained stable and she became more alert. Her respiration rate ranged from between 18/min and 22/min and her blood pressure and pulse remained stable. Her blood sugar was normal (3–6 mmol/litre) and her blood alcohol level was 125 mg alcohol/100 ml blood.

Session 1
This took place 4 days after Jane had taken the overdose. Jane attended with her daughter. The following sessions took place weekly.

Problem 4

Relationship with boy-friend.
Jane had not spoken to her boy-friend, although he had been in contact with her aunt and demanded that she return to him. Jane said that she had decided that she would leave her boy-friend permanently, but she was worried how he would react. A psychiatric social worker was suggested to advise on legal steps.

Problem 5

Feelings of helplessness.
Although still very tearful, Jane had had no further thoughts of taking an overdose.

Problem 7

Unsuitable accommodation.
Jane felt more relaxed staying with her aunt and stated that she would like to return to her parents. It was agreed that a social worker would join Jane and the therapist at the end of the next session.

Problem 9

Need for emotional support from parents.
Jane stated that she longed to return home to her parents. She found them more sympathetic and was able to discuss with them some of her difficulties in the past 2 years since leaving home. Her parents were relieved because Jane had talked to them about her problems, although Jane said they voiced some disappointment that she had not been able to approach them before the overdose.

Session 2

Problem 4

Relationship with boy-friend.
Jane's boy-friend had visited Jane at her parents and reluctantly agreed to a separation which he hoped would be only temporary. Her anxieties about separating were still evident, but Jane felt positive about life without him.

Problem 6

Social isolation.
It appeared that Jane's only relationships were with people older than herself, usually relatives. The therapist and Jane looked at how she could re-establish contacts with some old friends whom she had not seen since the birth of her daughter.

Problem 7

Unsuitable accommodation.
Jane agreed to longer-term work with the social worker to look at accommodation in the future. Jane felt that it was not realistic to return to live with her parents permanently.

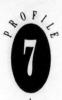
Problem 8

Anxiety about social service involvement.
The social worker explored how the relationship between Jane and the social services could be useful and discussed Jane's reservations and anxieties of social work allocation.

Problem 9

Relationship with parents.
Jane reported that staying with her parents was working out well. She was surprised at this and felt that it may not last for long.

Session 3

Problem 4

Relationship with boy-friend.
Jane expressed a feeling of emptiness and suggested that she was missing her boy-friend. She explained that, despite his behaviour, she still had some affection for him. She acknowledged that she was showing a normal reaction to her 'loss' and that this would lead to earlier resolution than if she bottled her feelings up.

Problem 5

Feelings of helplessness.
Jane had taken the initiative to contact her health visitor. The health visitor had visited Jane at her parents and reassured her that there appeared to be no problems with her daughter and that she would visit regularly. Taking this initiative was an important issue for Jane as she now felt that she was beginning to take responsibility for herself which boosted her self-esteem.

Problem 6

Social isolation.
Jane had visited two old friends who had welcomed her and seemed pleased to re-establish contact.

Problems 7 and 8

Accommodation problem and anxiety of social service involvement.
Jane would be seeing the social worker on a regular basis. Both the social worker and the health visitor had reassured her that there was no reason to take the baby away from her and that their help would be supportive.

Session 4
This was the final session with the therapist.

Problem 9

Relationship with parents.
Jane attended with both her parents and her aunt. She wanted to talk to her parents openly in the session. The therapist facilitated this discussion. Jane explained that she could not discuss her problems with her parents previously, mainly because she felt that as an 'adult' she could not return and ask for advice as a 'child' might. This prompted tears from both Jane and her mother which led them to talk about their roles in the family and how best they could help and support each other.

After Jane's parents and her aunt left the room, the therapist prompted Jane to reflect on the overdose and the changes that had occurred as a result. She was asked how she might cope with a similar crisis and responded as follows:

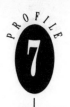

1. Maintain her relationship with her parents where problems could be discussed as they occur.
2. Continue to see her social worker and health visitor for support and practical advice.
3. Use open-access agencies, such as the Samaritans or A&E departments to prevent taking an overdose if a crisis should occur.

It was agreed that no further appointment was necessary but that she could contact the therapist in the event of future difficulties.

Answers to questions 1, 2 and 4

Problem 2

Question 1

The risks associated with a stomach wash-out are:

1. The risk of inserting the gastric tube into the lung.

Intervention
When the tube has been inserted, aspirate for stomach contents and test with blue litmus paper if unsure. If no aspirate is obtained, rapidly inject a small amount of air while auscultating over the gastric region. Bubbling should be heard.
2. The risk of aspirating stomach contents.

Interventions
a. Tilt head of trolley down.
b. Lie patient on left-hand side.
c. Have a large suction catheter (Yankaur) ready if patient vomits during the procedure.
d. If patient unrousable, infiltrate before starting wash-out, in presence of an anaesthetist.
3. The risk of the patient's panicking, causing her to be unable to breathe and so to fight the procedure.

Interventions
a. Fully explain the stomach wash-out beforehand, reassuring the patient that she will be able to breathe normally.
b. When the tube has been passed into the stomach, give the patient time to get used to the feeling and help her with her breathing before starting the wash-out.

Problem 3

Question 2

Expected outcome and interventions to prevent respiratory depression are that Jane's respiration rate will not fall below 16/min and that she will remain conscious and rousable.

Interventions
1. Monitor pulse, blood pressure and respiration rate ½ hourly while in A&E department.
2. Record level of consciousness and orientation.

3. Stomach wash-out. (Not indicated if only alcohol involved.)
4. Send blood sample for alcohol level 1 hour after ingestion.
5. Record blood glucose level using BM Stix.

Question 3

One further problem concerning Jane's family is the concern felt by her parents and her father's negative feelings towards her at present.

Cause
Lack of understanding about the reasons why Jane took the overdose, probably combined with feelings of guilt.

Expected outcome
That Jane's parents will understand the reasons why Jane took the overdose and will express a desire to help her.

Interventions
1. Explain to Jane the need for the nurse to talk to her parents and reassure them.
2. Ask Jane what she would like her parents to be told regarding her reasons for taking the overdose and if she would like to see them.
3. Talk to Jane's parents in private.
4. Explain to them the medical risks of the overdose and medical treatment—reassure them.
5. Determine and discuss their understanding of the reasoning behind the overdose.
6. Explain the need for their help and support.
7. Explain the later involvement of a social worker and health visitor to help Jane cope with the problems at home.

Problem 5

Question 4

Additional interventions to help Jane overcome her feelings of helplessness may include:

1. Provide time for Jane to look at her feelings of helplessness.
2. Help her to reflect on positive changes that she has activated in the past.
3. Provide details of self-help groups, such as Gingerbread.

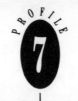

References

Brandon, S. (1976). Physical violence in the family—an overview. In: Borland, M. (ed.), *Violence in the family*, Manchester University Press, Manchester.

Brooking, J., and Minghella, E. (1987). Parasuicide. *Nursing Times*, **83** (21) 40–43.

Cosgriff, J. H., and Anderson, D. L. (1984). *The Practice of Emergency Care*, Lippincott, Philadelphia, Pennsylvania.

DHSS (1984). The management of deliberate self-harm. *Department of Health and Social Security Circular CMHN (84), LASL (84) 5*. HMSO, London.

Egan, G. (1982). *The Skilled Helper: Model, Skills and Methods for Effective Helping*, 2nd edn, Brooks/Cole, Monterey, California.

Hawton, K., and Catalan, J. (1987). *Attempted Suicide: A Practical Guide to Nature and Management*, 2nd edn, Oxford Medical Publications, Oxford.

Kreitman, N. (1977). *Parasuicide*, Wiley, London.

Macy, A. M. (1979). Preventing hepatotoxicity in acetaminophen overdose. *American Journal of Nursing*, **79**, 310–313.

Michell, J. R., *et al.* (1974). Acetaminophen-induced hepatic injury: protective role of glutathione in man and rationale for therapy. *Clinical Pharmacology and Therapeutics*, **16**, 676–684.

Morgan, H. G., Burns-Cox, C. T., Pocock, H., and Pottle, S. (1975). Deliberate self-harm: clinical and socio-economic characteristics of 368 patients. *British Journal of Psychiatry*, **126**, 564–574.

Rumack, B. H., and Matthews, H. (1975). Acetaminophen poisoning and toxicity. *Pediatrics*, **55**, 871–876.

Stanley, W. J. (1969). Attempted suicide and suicidal gestures. *British Journal of Preventive and Social Medicine*, **23**, 190–195.

Walsh, M. (1982). Patterns of drug overdose. *Nursing Times*, **78** (7), 275–278.

Walsh, M. (1985). *Accident and Emergency Nursing: A New Approach*, Heinemann, London.

Lynn Batehup

Recovery from a stroke:

Rehabilitation in the acute recovery stage

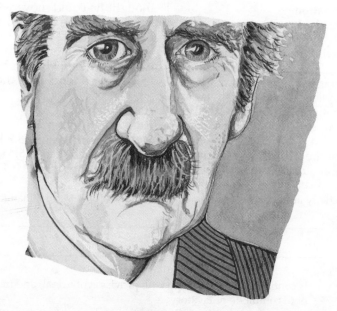

Because of their sudden helplessness, patients who have had a stroke feel great frustration at losing their independence and are most anxious about what the future might hold for them. Some of the physical and psychological problems of these patients are outlined. Identification of further difficulties and their causes and the appropriate interventions are required; the answers are given at the end of the chapter.

Patient profile

Mr Colin Freeman was admitted on August 19 to an acute medical ward with a left cerebrovascular accident and a right hemiplegia. On the day of admission, he had gone to the post office and, when coming out, he felt 'faint' and 'peculiar'. The next thing that he remembers is finding himself in the accident and emergency department of the local hospital. He was admitted to the ward in a drowsy state. The following assessment was carried out 2 weeks later.

Assessment information
Biographical and social information
Mr Freeman is 64 years old, married to his second wife with whom he lives in a second-floor maisonette. He has two grown-up children—an unmarried son, and a married daughter who both live away. Visits are fairly regular. He has not worked for 4 years and has diagnosed temporal lobe epilepsy controlled on medication. He had a fit the day before the onset of the stroke. Mrs Freeman does not have a job outside the home since

she had a hip operation 4 years ago. They share the daily chores.

Current health status
Mr Freeman realises that he has had a stroke, leaving him without movement down the right side of his body. He feels frustrated that recovery is slow and anxious about doing exercises as he says that he does not 'want to overdo it and cause more problems to himself'. However, he has fallen out of the chair and commode on two occasions because he thought he could move without help. He is feeling miserable about what the future holds for him. Mr and Mrs Freeman have been told that the maisonette will not be suitable for his predicted mobility. Mrs Freeman also feels despondent about the future.

Assessment
Eating and drinking
Mr Freeman weighs 66.7 kg and is 5 ft 3 in tall; so he is about 3.2–6.4 kg overweight. He has a good appetite. Mr Freeman was seen

Table 8.1 Activity and mobility assessment and the scores for Mr Freeman (scoring criteria on p. 74)

Activity		Score
Self-care activities		
Continence	Is continent but needs help with provision of urinal, and transfer onto commode or lavatory	3
Grooming	Can use left hand to wash face and hand, and to clean teeth. Needs help with provision of water and washing utensils	3
Bathing	Transfers into and out of the bath with one helper using mechanical hoist. Can wash a large part of his body	3
Use of lavatory	Transfers with one helper	3
Feeding	Needs help to cut food but can be independent if special rocker knife is used	2
Dressing	Needs help from one person	3
Mobility activities		
Sitting up in bed	Needs help from two people in order to prevent shoulder damage	3
Transfer	Needs help from one person	3
Standing	Unable to extend hip or to lock knee	3
Level walking	Unable, even with help	4

by the dietitian, started on a reducing, high-fibre diet and asked to reduce his salt intake. He eats and enjoys all the food given to him and has no difficulty with chewing or swallowing. He does need help with cutting up meat. He wears dentures which still fit well.

Communicating

Mr Freeman's speech is rapid and fluent with no obvious difficulties. His reading ability is still intact, and he appears to have no visual field defects. He is right handed and finds writing difficult.

Emotional state

This is obviously labile. He cries easily. He starts to sob silently with his shoulders moving up and down during conversations. The crying seems to correspond to mentions of his wife, home, dog and future. He is an outgoing friendly person who seems to enjoy talking to people.

Working and playing

Mr Freeman has not worked for 4 years but was a plastics moulder until he felt that the frequency of his fits was becoming unpredictable. He collects an invalidity pension and does not appear unhappy about not working. His recreational pastimes are few and include listening to the radio and music, some television and reading the daily paper. He walks his dog three times a day. 'Has a quiet life.'

Activity and mobility assessment

This is shown in Table 8.1. A description and scoring criteria are included in the evaluation section.

Problems, expected outcomes, and interventions

Plans for stroke patients should be reviewed regularly.

Problem 1

Loss of voluntary movement of the right limbs and trunk with abnormal levels of muscle tone (some flaccidity and some spasticity). Possible malalignment of the shoulder joint.

Cause

Probably thromboembolic infarction, causing brain damage to motor and sensory centres, and hyperexcitability of spinal stretch reflexes.

Expected outcomes

1. For patient to maintain existing range of joint movement on both sides of the body, and to avoid joint contracture.
2. Absence of damage to vulnerable joints until some return of voluntary movement.
3. An absence of undue increase in spasticity in the affected limbs.
4. Patient will experience stimulation to the affected side.
5. The patient and carers to feel informed and participate in all activities when able to.

Question 1

On a separate sheet of paper, can you suggest a list of interventions that would result in meeting (or trying to meet) these expected outcomes?

Question 2

Can you also indicate the probable pattern of limb spasticity that might occur in an untreated patient?

Problem 2

Impaired mobility and postural balance mechanism. Unable to use his right arm and hand, or to support himself when upright.

Cause
Cerebral infarction, causing damage to motor and sensory nerves which supply the right side of the body.

Expected outcomes
1. He will be able to roll and move himself in bed, and to sit up from lying, helped by one person and then unaided. This may take a week or two.
2. He will transfer from bed to chair and back with the help of one person. This may take a week.
3. He will use remaining function to perform self-care activities without becoming tired or frustrated.
4. His carer will learn and participate to her level of ability.

Interventions
In consultation with the physiotherapist, patient and carer, plan a retraining programme:

1. Mr Freeman to move from sitting on the bed unsupported—sitting balance.
2. For the transfer technique, he will be assisted by one person, using a standard technique.
3. Assistance with self-care activities will be given but should allow the patient to participate to the level of his capacities without becoming tired. Space activities to include rest periods.
4. Teach and involve the chief carer in all activities when possible.

The programme for restoration of mobility should follow a logical developmental sequence. Walking does not start until balance and some control of hip, knee and foot have been attained.

Question 3

On a separate sheet of paper, can you suggest any other problems that this patient may be experiencing? Make a list with their cause, expected outcomes, and interventions.

Rationale

Positioning and handling

Immediately following a stroke, the affected limbs usually show a reduction in postural muscle tone—flaccid paralysis. However, gradually over a period of weeks or months, it is seen that a large number of patients show an increase in muscle tone—spasticity. The distribution of spasticity follows a characteristic pattern in a large number of patients (Twitchell, 1951). However, some patients' flaccidity persists, especially in the upper limb. The reasons for this are poorly understood (Rankin, 1957), and the prognosis for return of useful function is poor.

According to Bobath (1979), abnormal patterns of postural tone can be avoided or at least minimised by positioning the limbs correctly. Lack of movement of the affected limbs will soon result in joint contractures, a shortening and thickening of muscle, tendons, ligaments and capsule surrounding a joint. Range of motion in an immobilised joint may decline in as little as 3 days (Sharpless, 1982).

Contractures cause pain, increased spasticity and significant impairment in function and can be avoided by carrying out a passive range of motion exercises two to three times a day. Nurses and carers can be shown how to do this without causing pain or damage.

Retraining mobility

According to Bobath (1979), movement for the hemiplegic person is difficult for three reasons: the patient feels divided into two halves with the one having nothing to do with the other; postural muscle tone of the two sides is different with a mixture of spasticity and flaccidity; the patient no longer knows how to move. He has to relearn how to turn over in bed, how to sit up, how to lie down, how to stand and how to walk. He has little or no balance and is always fearful of falling to the affected side.

Johnstone (1977) describes a stepwise programme of retraining which follows a developmental pattern, starting with bed movements, rolling, sitting up and sitting balance. This progresses to transfer techniques, standing balance and eventually walking. These activities have been described by Parry and Eales (1976), Batehup (1983) and Myco (1983).

Every movement that the nurse does with the patient is new to him. He has to learn to adjust and cope with each new situation. He should not be moved hurriedly, nor be passive when being moved from one position to another. He should be given the opportunity actively to follow the movements done with him (Bobath, 1979).

Post-stroke complications

Shoulder malalignment and subluxation

Subluxation of the shoulder after stroke has been recognised for some time (Miglietta *et al.*, 1959) and may vary from a few millimetres of malalignment to moderate and severe subluxation (Smith *et al.*, 1982). A study by Smith *et al.* (1982) found that, in a group of 46 patients with complete paralysis of the arm, 60% showed some degree of malalignment.

During the stage of flaccid paralysis the gravitational pull of the affected arm on the shoulder muscles causes stretching of the joint capsule. Studies show that malalignment usually occurs during this period and is by no means always a consequence of prolonged paralysis or disuse (Smith *et al.*, 1982). Problems with the shoulder can occur under three circumstances (Mulley, 1985): incorrect positioning and handling—leaving the arm unsupported or pulling at it; overstrenuous arm movement; failure to keep the shoulder mobilised with passive movements.

Deep vein thrombosis (DVT)

It is unusual for stroke patients *not* to develop DVT in the paralysed leg in the early stages of their illness (Warlow *et al.*, 1972). DVT can be detected within 48 hours of the stroke, and most patients develop this complication within 10 days (McCarthy *et al.*, 1979). Usual signs and symptoms of DVT are not useful for detecting post-stroke DVT, and pyrexia

may be the only sign (Murray *et al.*, 1979). All oedematous paralysed legs should be noted and not ascribed to immobility, even when calf pain is absent. The use of accurately measured anti-embolism stockings has not been shown to prevent emboli development after a stroke but might reduce oedema (Mulley, 1985).

Depression

Depression is common after a stroke, with a recent study (Robinson *et al.*, 1982) finding a third of patients examined depressed and, furthermore, it is seldom treated and often not even diagnosed (Mulley, 1985). There are two possible causes put forward: that it is a failure to adapt to stroke and that counselling may help; that in some cases it is the effect of reduced neurotransmitter levels, specially when damage is to the frontal area of the brain (Lipsey *et al.*, 1984).

A major difficulty is in spotting depression in stroke patients, for problems in communication and perception may mask symptoms. Nurses and carers need to be aware of the possibility that this is happening.

Emotionalism

Excessive or inappropriate weepiness or laughter can occur after any stroke. There are different degrees of emotionalism (Parish and James, 1982): laughing or crying when any attempt is made to talk to the patient—emotional incontinence; crying is provoked when conversation is about home, relatives, future outcomes—emotional lability; finally, catastrophic reactions, a combination of anger, frustration and depression, resulting in an emotional outburst of sobbing and hopelessness. A positive and understanding atmosphere is necessary for rehabilitation, and this is even more important in helping the patient to overcome these and other psychological sequelae (Rankin, 1957; Sharpless, 1982).

Evaluation

The average stay in hospital for the stroke patient is about 3 months. It is probably necessary to review the plan weekly or more frequently if problems are of a short-term nature. Table 8.2 shows the three stages of recovery from stroke, and some general areas for evaluation over time. It is useful to use some form of repeatable assessment such as that described here (Tables 8.3 and 8.4) by Parish and James (1982).

This is only one form of assessment of many described in the literature, but it has been shown to be useful in assessing and evaluating recovery over time in individual stroke patients.

Table 8.2 The three stages of stroke recovery

Early stage up to 3 weeks
There may be perceptual and sensory impairment
Feeding and drinking impairment may be noticed
Elimination impairment is possible
Correct positioning is essential
Passive exercise is essential

Table 8.2 (continued)

Middle stage up to 3 months
Correct positioning is of importance
Contractures may be apparent
Retraining in balance and co-ordination should begin
Ambulation should be started
Start to retrain in functional activities including dressing, grooming,
  feeding and elimination
Mood and emotions vary
Knowledge and skills levels of patient and carers should be assessed
Planning should be started for future lifestyle changes, for example
  attention should be given to matters such as the person's job, his
  income, the suitability of his home

Later stage up to 2 years
Mobility with or without aids should be obvious
Maintaining achieved levels of function and mobility when home should
  be the aim
Social integration should be encouraged
Sexual function may be resumed
Continuing support of carers is essential

Table 8.3 Activity assessment: activities and definitions

Activity	Definition
Self-care activities	
Continence	Able to control bladder and bowels by day and night
Grooming	Wash face and hands, clean teeth, comb hair, shave, wash rest of the body
Bathing	Get into and out of the bath and wash all over body
Use of lavatory	Use the lavatory (or commode) and adjust clothing
Feeding	Cut up and eat food
Dressing	Get and put on clothes
	Undress
	Manage fasteners, etc.
Mobility activities	
Sitting up in bed	Move from lying to sitting position
Transfer	Move out of bed or chair onto feet and sit or lie down after standing (or into or out of a wheelchair if wheelchair mobile)
Standing	Stand with both feet flat on the floor
Level walking	Unaided on level floor

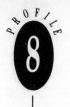
Table 8.4 Mobility assessment: four levels of assistance

Scoring criteria	Score
Able to perform the activity without help from another person or with aids	1
Able to carry out the activity without help from another person, but with a physical aid if necessary	2
Able to perform the activity with or without an aid but requires help from another person—could be verbal or physical assistance	3
Complete inability to contribute to the performance of the activity in any way, even with assistance	4

Answers to questions 1, 2 and 3

Problem 1

Question 1

Interventions that would help the patient to meet the expected outcomes listed for a patient who has loss of voluntary movement of the right limbs and trunk, with abnormal levels of the muscle tone would be:

1. Incorporate teaching activities for patient and carers into all interventions.

2. Nurse or carers to carry out passive movements and range of joint exercises two to three times a day.
3. Position limbs in antireflex patterns (antispasticity positions) (Table 8.5).
4. Handle limbs and patient to prevent damage to joints, especially the affected shoulder.
5. Help the patient from the affected side. Orient the patient to the affected side with touch and other stimulation.
6. Use a bed cradle.

Problem 1

Question 2

The 'typical spastic' hemiplegic pattern that might occur in an untreated patient is as follows:

1. *Head*. Turned to the affected side.

2. *Neck*. Laterally flexed to the affected side.
3. *Shoulder*. Retracted—pulled downwards and backwards.
4. *Arm*. Turned inwards and held into the side of the body.
5. *Elbow*. Flexed.

6. *Fingers*. Flexed, with the thumb across the palm of the hand.
7. *Trunk*. Flexed to the affected side.
8. *Leg*. Extended and rolled outwards.
9. *Foot*. Usually with toes pointing downwards and tending to turn inwards.

Some patients, especially the very old, may be seen with a flaccid upper limb, and a tendency to flexion of the lower limbs, that is flexed hip and knee and the leg abducted.

Table 8.5 Evaluation criteria for positioning stroke patients

Limb	Criteria
Lying on the affected side	
Head, neck, trunk	Elongated and in a straight line. Trunk to the waist can be supported on a pillow
Shoulder	Pulled forwards
Arm	Out straight with palm of hand facing upwards. Do not place anything in the palm of the hand
Leg	Hip and knee slightly bent. The upper limb supported on a pillow. Do not place anything against the bottom of the affected foot
Lying on the unaffected side	
Head, neck, trunk	Elongated and in a straight line
Shoulder	Pulled forwards, with the arm supported on a pillow
Arm	Out straight with palm facing down, and the fingers extended
Leg	Hip and knee slightly bent, supported on a pillow
Sitting in a chair	
Head	Facing to the front
Neck, trunk	In a straight line with each other
Shoulder, arm	Forward at the shoulder with the arm extended supported on a pillow on a table, or with fingers of both hands clasped, and supported on a table in front
Hips, knees, ankles, feet	Should all be at right angles, with the feet flat on the floor. Should be sitting well back in an upright chair. Avoid too much padding out with pillows or an air ring

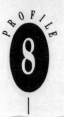

Question 3

Another problem that Mr Freeman might be having is emotional lability. He has frequent episodes of crying which may or may not be provoked by an encounter which has sentimental connections.

Cause

Organic brain dysfunction related to cerebral infarction.

Expected outcome

Should have an insight into the reasons for these outbursts and feel some relief from the worry about them.

Interventions

1. Provide a positive and supportive environment.
2. Explain to the patient and carers that this behaviour is related to the brain damage and is as much an effect of the stroke as are the paralysed limbs. It is not a sign of psychiatric disease and will gradually resolve with time.
3. Emphasise that it is not the fault of the carers or anybody else.

In Mr Freeman's case, the crying episodes stopped completely within 4 weeks.

A further problem is his potential depressive state. Mr Freeman has expressed feelings of worthlessness and low self-esteem. He is also anxious and unhappy.

Causes

Despair, perceived loss of control, loss of dignity, loss of function and fear of another stroke.

Expected outcomes

1. Will have an insight into the possibility that this problem arises, and some awareness of the signs and behaviours that could be present.
2. Will feel able to talk about his feelings and fears and anxieties.

Interventions

1. Make time to listen and talk, and to develop a trusting relationship with the patient and carers.
2. Having a knowledge of risk indicators for depression in stroke patients, so that carers and nurses can monitor them:
   a. Patients who were previously active, and now feel helpless and fear permanent disability.
   b. Patients with left hemisphere frontal lobe infarctions; feelings of anxiety, hopelessness, irritability; feelings of anxiety, hopelessness, irritability.
   c. Patients with sleep disturbances, appetite disturbance, weight loss, constipation.
   d. Patients with loss of interest, loss of energy and social withdrawal.

References

Batehup, L. (1983). How teaching can help the stroke patient's recovery. In: Wilson-Barnett, J. (ed.), *Patient Teaching*, Churchill Livingstone, Edinburgh.

Bobath, B. (1979). *Adult Hemiplegia: Evaluation and Treatment*, Heinemann Medical Books, London.

Johnstone, M. (1977). *The Stroke Patient: Principles of Rehabilitation*. Churchill Livingstone, Edinburgh.

Lipsey, J. R., Robinson, R. G., Pearlson, G. D., Rao, K., and Price T. R. (1984). Nortryptylline treatment of post-stroke depression: a double blind study. *The Lancet*, **1**, 297–300.

McCarthy, S. T., Robertson, D., Turner, J. J., and Hawkey, C. J. (1979). Low dose heparin as a prophylaxis against deep vein thrombosis after acute stroke. *The Lancet*, **2**, 800–801.

Miglietta, O., Lewitan, A., and Rogoff, J. B. (1959). Subluxation of the shoulder in hemiplegic patients. *New York State Journal of Medicine*, **59**, 457–460.

Mulley, G. P. (1985). *Practical Management of the Stroke Patient*, Croom Helm, London.

Murray, H. W., Ellis, G. C., Blumenthal, D. S., and Sos, T. A. (1979). Fever and pulmonary embolism. *American Journal of Medicine*, **67**, 232–235.

Myco, F. (1983). *Nursing Care of the Hemiplegic Stroke Patient*, Harper and Row, London.

Parish, G. J., and James, D. W. (1982). A method of evaluating the level of independence during the rehabilitation of the disabled. *Rheumatology and Rehabilitation*, **21**, 107–114.

Parry, A., and Eales, C. (1976). The ambulant stroke patient. *Nursing Times*, **72**, 1726–1730.

Rankin, J. (1957). Cerebrovascular accidents in patients over the age of 60. Prognosis. *Scottish Medical Journal*, **2**, 200–215.

Robinson, R. G., Thomas, R., and Price, T. R. (1982). Post-stroke disorders: a follow-up study of 103 patients. *Stroke*, **13**, 635–640.

Sharpless, J. W. (1982). *Mossman's, A Problem Oriented Approach to Stroke Rehabilitation*, Charles C. Thomas, Springfield, Virginia.

Smith, R. G., Cruickshank, J. G., Dunbar, S., and Akhtar, A. J. (1982). Malalignment of the shoulder after stroke. *British Medical Journal*, **284**, 1224–1226.

Twitchell, T. E. (1951). The restoration of motor function after hemiplegia in man. *Brain*, **74**, 443–480.

Warlow, C., Ogstone, D., and Douglas, A. S. (1972). Venous thrombosis following strokes. *The Lancet*, **1**, 1305–1306.

Sally Glen

A patient who has had a lobectomy:

Planning in the acute post-operative period

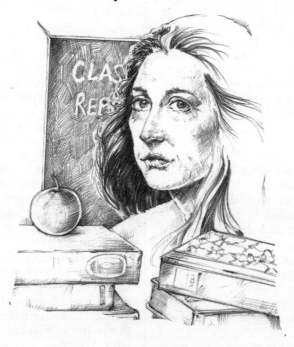

Ann Gates was admitted to hospital when breathlessness and recurrent chest pains were preventing her from functioning adequately both at work and leisure. Subsequently an operation was carried out to remove a lobe of her right lung. This chapter provides the assessment data, problems identified and intervention carried out after this operation; answers are given at the end of the chapter.

Patient profile

Ms Ann Gates is a 41-year-old teacher who lives with her girl-friend Liz Edwards in a house which they own jointly. They have lived together for the past 5 years. Ann spends most of her free time going to the cinema and theatre and reading.

Assessment information
Previous health
Ann has had the usual childhood illnesses, but none that could account for her bronchiectasis. This developed as a result of right lower lobe pneumonia with a streptococcal lung abscess in 1979. At that time, she was admitted to hospital with a 1-week history of 'flu' and shortness of breath with a wheeze. This was treated with antibiotics and postural drainage. Since then she has been fit enough to work but has been persistently troubled with breathlessness and recurrent chest infections.

Current health
Ann's exercise tolerance has become gradually impaired by breathlessness and she is unable to walk up gradients without becoming dyspnoeic. This resulted in her having a bilateral bronchogram as a day-care patient in order to reassess the condition of her lungs. This revealed incomplete filling of the right lower lobe, suggesting the presence of bronchiectasis. A bronchoscopy showed no abnormality. Pulmonary function tests were also performed. The results were as in Table 9.1.

When the results of the examination were known, the consultant thoracic surgeon explained to Ann that she had an infected lobe of her right lung and advised her to have it removed. The doctor also explained that she could not guarantee any great improvement following the operation.

Assessment
Psychological safety
Ann relies on her girl-friend Liz for support. Her mother and married sister who has two children live 45 min away. Ann talks on the telephone to her mother twice a week, and has Sunday dinner with the family about once a month.

Breathing
During Ann's introduction to the lay-out of the ward, it became obvious that she became breathless at the slightest exertion. Before coming into hospital Ann was having a Salbutamol inhaler two inhalations four times a day, and a beclamethasone inhaler, also four times a day. This was to improve her respiratory function as much as possible. Ann does not smoke. Sputum culture proved negative. Her temperature was 36.8 °C, her blood pressure 130/85 mmHg and her pulse 80/min (Blackburn and Cebenka, 1980).

Eating and drinking
24-hour diet recall.
Breakfast: banana, coffee.
Lunch: tuna fish and wholemeal bread, one apple, one orange, coffee.
Supper: pasta, one serving of ice cream, one to two pieces of fruit, two to three glasses of wine, coffee.

Ann says that she is a vegetarian, although she will eat fish.

Table 9.1 Pulmonary function tests

	Result (litres)	Result (%)	Predicted (litres)	Predicted (%)
Forced expiratory volume in 1 s	2.35	44	3.6	65
Forced vital capacity	5.30		4.6	115

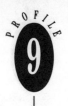

Sleeping
Ann usually sleeps 7–8 hours a night. She goes to bed about 11.00 pm and awakes at 6.45 am. She usually falls asleep easily and manages to sleep, as long as she has three pillows.

Eliminating
Ann suffers from chronic constipation which she treats with over-the-counter laxatives. She has a bowel movement once every 3–4 days. Urine culture and examination proved negative.

Communicating
Ann expressed concern that the operation was 'futile'. She states that her illness was increasingly restricting her life.

Personal cleansing
Ann has patchy areas of dry skin on her legs and arms. States that she has a 'tendency to eczema'. She does not use soap on her skin and instead uses aqueous cream to moisturise her skin, and Emulsificans in the bath.

Mobilising
Her exercise tolerance is impaired by breath-lessness, and she is unable to walk up gradients without becoming very dyspnoeic.

Expressing sexuality
Ann states that she has had a stable relation-ship with her girl-friend Liz for 6 years. She says that their relationship has changed since she has become unwell over the past year. She hopes that their relationship will change for the better after the operation (Pogoncheff, 1979; Pettyjohn, 1979).

Problems, expected outcomes, and interventions

Pre-operative care plan
The pre-operative care plan is concerned with dealing with Ann's knowledge deficit re-lated to the pre- and post-operative regime. It would be expected that, following the nursing interventions, Ann would be able to relate the routine concerning her pre- and post-operative care and demonstrate post-operative breathing and coughing exercises. The remainder of this plan will concentrate on the post-operative period.

Problem 1

Potential risk of lung collapse related to air collection in the chest cavity, and potential risk of bleeding into the chest cavity.

Cause
Possible collection of blood and exudate in the pleura following surgery.

Expected outcomes
1. That blood and exudate does not re-main in the pleura.
2. That the pulse rate remains within normal limits 85/min.
3. That blood loss via the drains will be in the region of 50 ml in 24 hours.

Interventions
1. Check the intercostal drains to see whether the fluid is swinging and bubbling.
2. Monitor blood pressure, pulse, respira-tory rate and character.

Problem 2

Potential risk of chest infection related to post-operative lung consolidation.

Cause
Shallow breathing post-operatively related to pain.

Expected outcomes
1. That the sputum remains clear and colourless.
2. That Ann will be able to expectorate and take deep breaths without discomfort.

Interventions
1. Give oxygen via the MC mask at 5 l/min.
2. Use a 'preventive approach' (Jacox, 1979; McCaffery, 1980):
   a. Give medication before activity, for example physiotherapy.
   b. Assess the respiratory rate before giving analgesia.
   c. Ask Ann to request pain relief before the pain is severe.
3. Teach Ann how to support the wound when coughing.
4. The physiotherapist to visit at 4-hourly intervals for coughing and expectoration of sputum. Also for deep breathing and shoulder exercises.
5. To carry out deep breathing and coughing at 2-hourly intervals throughout the day until 10.00 pm.

Question 1

On a separate sheet of paper, can you identify any other actual or potential problems relevant to this patient?

Evaluation

Problem 1

Potential lung collapse.
1. The drainage from each bottle was recorded every ½ hour to start with.
2. The following day the underwater seal bottles were changed. Drainage for the first 24 hours was 340 ml. Chest x-rays showed chest expansion.
3. The second day the drainage from both underwater seal bottles was minimal and oscillation of the fluid had ceased. The two intercostal tubes were removed.
4. Observation of blood pressure, temperature, pulse and respirations were recorded ½-hourly to start with. After midnight, they were recorded hourly. After this, observations were gradually reduced to 4-hourly.

Problem 2

Potential chest infection.
1. Oxygen was discontinued after 3 hours as her colour was pink and respiration had settled from 28/min to 18/min.
2. After giving analgesia the nurse returned at ½ hour to assess its effectiveness.
3. She was able to deep-breathe, expectorate and participate with the physiotherapist without discomfort.
4. Temperature was monitored.

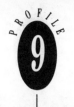
Rationale

Bronchiectasis is a dilation of the bronchi or bronchial tubes. Secretions accumulate, and chronic infection causes persistent cough and purulent sputum. This condition occurs in approximately 1:1000 of the population and in most cases develops in childhood.

The objectives of Ms Gate's pre-operative care were:

1. To ascertain her functional reserve to see whether she could survive the operation.
2. To ensure her optimal condition for surgery and recovery.

Consequently a range of tests were carried out to determine her pre-operative condition, and to assess her physical assets and liabilities. These included pulmonary function tests to decide whether the contemplated resection would leave sufficient functional lung tissue, and blood gases to provide a more complete picture of the functional capacity of the lung. In addition, other tests were carried out to provide a baseline for comparison during the post-operative period. These include chest x-ray, electrocardiogram, serum creatinine to assess renal function and blood electrolytes, and serum proteins.

Pre-operative nursing intervention

Ms Gates was informed as to what to expect in the post-operative period. This includes the possible presence of chest tubes, drainage bottles and the use of oxygen to help with breathing. The importance of frequent turning to promote drainage of lung secretions was explained. In addition, Ms Gates was instructed in the technique of coughing in order to bring up secretions and warned that this might prove to be uncomfortable. She was taught to splint her incision with her hands or a pillow.

Psychological support

Several days were allocated to Ms Gates' pre-operative preparation. This provided time for her primary nurse to talk with her. By listening, the nurse discovered how she really felt about her illness and the proposed treatment. Ms Gates revealed significant reactions such as fear of death because of chronic respiratory disease. The primary nurse tried to help Ms Gates to overcome many of her fears, and to use her intellectual functions in order to cope with the stress of surgery. This can be done by using the following strategy:

1. By correcting any false impressions.
2. By offering reassurance about the capability of the surgical team.
3. By telling Ms Gates that her incision will hold.
4. By dealing honestly with questions about pain, discomfort and her treatment.

The management and control of pain began before surgery by informing Ms Gates that she herself could overcome many post-operative problems by following routines related to deep breathing, coughing and turning.

Post-operative nursing intervention

The goals of the patient are:

1. Improvement of breathing.
2. Relief of pain and discomfort.
3. Relief of anxiety.

A thoracotomy incision is used when the pleura is entered. The involved lung collapses and, after the lobe is removed, the remaining lobe of the lung is re-expanded. Frequently, two chest catheters are inserted for drainage. The upper one is for removal of air, and the lower one is for drainage of fluid. The chest tubes are connected to underwater seal drainage bottles. There may be some further bleeding and exudation from the chest wall and mediastinum. Every effort is made to prevent this blood and exudate from remaining in the pleura, as it would eventually become organised into fibrous tissue and impair the residual lung. After the operation, the major nursing objective is to restore

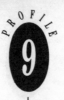
normal cardiopulmonary function as quickly as possible. This is done by:

1. Maintaining a patent airway.
2. Providing for maximum expansion of the remaining lung tissue.
3. Recognising early signs and symptoms of complications.
4. Providing supportive and rehabilitative measures.

Excessive secretions will produce airway obstruction, causing air in the alveoli distal to the obstruction to become absorbed and the lung to collapse. Atelectasis, pneumonia and respiratory failure may follow. Therefore, secretions must be suctioned. Most post-operative lobectomy patients are given humidified oxygen because their ventilation mechanism is impaired primarily as a result of pain and splinting of the operative side. The character and depth of respirations and the patient's colour are important criteria in evaluating the adequacy of lung expansion. The heart rate and rhythm are monitored as major arrhythmic episodes are common after thoracic and cardiac surgery. An arterial line is maintained to facilitate frequent monitoring of blood gases, serum electrolytes, haemoglobin, haematocrit values and arterial pressures.

The patient must be encouraged to cough effectively, since ineffective coughing will lead to exhaustion and retention of secretions, which can in turn lead to atelectasis and pneumonia. Pain can lead to post-operative complications if it reduces the patient's ability to cough and breath deeply. This may limit chest expansion so that effective ventilation is decreased.

Discharge planning and patient education
Before going home, it is advisable to give the following advice and information:

1. The patient should be aware that there is some intercostal pain for a period of time. This can be relieved by local heat and oral analgesia.
2. She should continue with deep-breathing exercises for several weeks at home.
3. She should practise good body alignment in front of a full-length mirror.
4. She should avoid lifting more than 20 lb until complete healing. This is up to 6 months.
5. Stop any activity that causes fatigue or increases shortness of breath.
6. She should stay away from respiratory irritants such as smoke, fumes and high air pollution.
7. Have an annual influenza injection if prescribed.
8. Attend follow-up out-patient appointments.

Answers to question 1

Problem 3

Potential risk of wound and drain site infection.

Cause
Possible colonisation and infection by micro-organisms from the patient's own flora; micro-organisms present during operation; micro-organisms present in the ward environment or personnel.

Expected outcomes
1. Absence of redness or swelling along the suture line or drain sites.
2. Healing by first intention within 10 days.

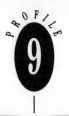
Interventions
1. Leave the main dressing intact.
2. Replace dressing around the drains only if soiled.
3. Monitor temperature for pyrexia.
4. Monitor for pain and discomfort.

Evaluation
On the tenth post-operative day the sutures were removed. It was noticed that part of the suture line was red and painful. Following probing of the wound by the doctor, there was a large discharge of pus which was sent for culture and sensitivity. The report showed that there was a *Staphylococcus aureus* infection sensitive to flucloxacillin. Antibiotics were prescribed.

Problem 4

Disturbance to self-concept.

Cause
Impairment of respiratory function.

Expected outcome
Ann will be able to demonstrate confidence in her ability to accomplish what she desires.

Interventions
1. Establish a trusting relationship with Ann.
2. Encourage her to express her feelings about the way that she feels, thinks or views herself.
3. Encourage her to ask questions about her health problems, treatment and prognosis.
4. Clarify any misconceptions that she has about herself, her care or care givers.
5. Avoid negative criticisms.

Evaluation
It should be possible to evaluate Ann's feelings about herself from her verbal statements and from her mood and general disposition/behaviour.

Problem 5

Potential impairment of skin integrity.

Cause
Post-operative immobility.

Expected outcomes
1. That the skin over pressure points remains intact.
2. An absence of redness or soreness.

Interventions
1. Assess Ann using the Norton score (Williams, 1972; Gruis and Innes, 1976).
2. Encourage range of motion exercise to increase blood flow.
3. Promote optimal circulation when in bed by turning every 2 hours or more if any red areas.

4. Position in normal or neutral position with body weight evenly distributed.
5. When moving Ann in bed, lift clear of the surface. Do not pull or slide skin surfaces.

Evaluation

The condition of body areas at risk such as elbows, heels, sacrum, scapula, ischia, ears and trochanter should be observed for erythema and blanching and should be felt for warmth and tissue sponginess.

References

Blackburn, N. A., and Cebenka, D. L. (1980). Holding your respiratory assessment technique. *Registered Nurse*, **43** (5), 28–33.

Gruis, M., and Innes, B. (1976). Assessment: essential to prevent pressure sores. *American Journal of Nursing*, **16**, 1762–1764.

Jacox, A. L. (1979). Assessing pain. *American Journal of Nursing*, **79**, 895–900.

McCaffery, M. (1980). *Nursing Management of The Patient with Pain*, Lippincot, Philadelphia, Pennsylvania.

Pettyjohn, R. D. (1979). Health care of the gay individual. *Nursing Forum*, **17**, 367–371.

Pogoncheff, E. (1979). The gay patient—what not to do. *Registered Nurse*, **42**, 46–48.

Williams, A. (1972). A study of factors contributing to skin breakdown. *Nursing Research*, **21**, 238–243.

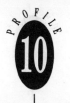

Jenifer Wilson-Barnett

A patient with heart failure:

Planning care for a successful recovery

The case of Celia Jones, who was admitted to hospital to control her heart failure and to treat a leg ulcer, is considered. The background information required for planning her care is given and three nursing problems are identified with their causes, expected outcomes and the interventions. Some other expected outcomes and interventions as well as other problems need to be identified; the answers are at the end of the chapter.

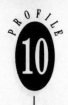
Patient profile

Mrs Celia Jones, aged 73, was finally admitted to hospital on the advice of her general practitioner, in an attempt to control her heart failure and to treat her leg ulcer. For 3 years, she has suffered intermittently from pulmonary and systemic oedema and recently complained of increasing tiredness and weakness. She has had two previous admissions to the same ward.

Assessment information
Biographical and social information
Mrs Jones has been a widow for 6 years and lives alone in a flat quite near to the hospital. Her only daughter lives 100 miles away with her husband and three teenage children. Several neighbours are friendly and helpful to Mrs Jones. She has a home help twice a week. Usually she is a talkative sociable lady.

Current and previous health status
Mrs Jones has been deteriorating for several weeks and realises that she is getting weaker. She is grateful and relieved to be admitted for treatment and rest. She is irritated by her leg ulcer which 'refuses' to heal. The district nursing sister has been calling once a week to dress the ulcer and to help Mrs Jones to shower. Present medications include tabs. digoxin 62.5 µg daily, and frusemide 40 mg daily and slow release potassium.

Mrs Jones suffered from rheumatic fever at the age of 13 which caused residual mitral valvular stenosis. This was not treated as it did not cause symptoms until Mrs Jones was in her sixties when atrial fibrillation developed. She has had a leg ulcer previously which took 3 months to heal, and two bouts of bronchitis in the past 10 days.

Assessment
Eating and drinking
Mrs Jones weighs 55 kg, and is 5 ft 4 in tall. Muscle wasting is evident and lower limb oedema obvious.

She suffers from indigestion and can tolerate only very small quantities. She eats small amounts of chicken and mashed potatoes, or occasionally fish. Although she is thirsty, Mrs Jones is reluctant to drink much because of fluid retention. Her skin is dry with little elasticity.

Eliminating
Constipation is a problem for Mrs Jones and she is passing small quantities of urine, infrequently.

Communicating
Understanding the disease Mrs Jones has learned that her heart is weak. She has fluid inside her lungs which prevents adequate oxygen from being absorbed, resulting in 'circulation problems' and 'breathlessness'.

She is very willing to talk about her illness and to expose her ulcer. She jokes a lot and seems easy to talk to.

Working and playing
Mrs Jones has been able to prepare her own food and to do the dusting. Lately, however, she has felt less able to do more than sit in her chair with her leg elevated. Her favourite pastime is watching television and chatting with her friend 'over the way'. She has a pension and this seems to be adequate to pay her rent and bills.

Sleeping
She manages to sleep for about 6 hours as long as she has three pillows. Lately she has noticed a tendency to 'drop off' in her chair at times throughout the day.

Personal cleansing
She has help for her weekly shower and relies on a daily wash at the basin at other times. Her lower right leg is covered with a plastic bag for this.

Mrs Jones has an ulcer on the right outer leg just above the external malleolus (size, 30 mm × 45 mm). It is not infected at present. It contains some necrotic tissue, and there is slight oozing of clear fluid.

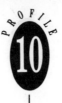

Breathing

Mrs Jones is breathless while sitting at rest in the chair. She is also using accessory muscles of respiration. Her respiratory rate is 40/min, her pulse 88 and irregular, her apex beat 108 and her blood pressure 120/60 mmHg.

Problems, expected outcomes, and interventions

Problem 1

Breathless at rest and when talking; cyanosed and cold; respiratory rate of 40/min.

Cause 1
1. Pulmonary oedema related to increased vascular pressures.
2. Poor airway clearance related to fluid accumulation in alveoli and bronchioles, and poor cough associated with weakness and fatigue.
3. Impaired gas exchange related to pulmonary oedema.

Expected outcomes
1. Respiratory rate decreased to 20/min in 3 days.
2. Demonstrates effective breathing pattern and coughing.
3. Able to talk with ease and comfort.
4. Achieve safe and comfortable mobility by 7 days.
5. Pulse regular and within normal limits in 3 days.

Interventions
1. Monitor pulse, blood pressure and apex beat twice daily.
2. Ensure that anti-arrhythmic and inotropic drugs are taken as prescribed. Monitor for side effects. Teach patient about their action and possible side-effects.
3. Teach and supervise lower limb exercises to prevent venous stasis.
4. Position in bed or chair to assist expiratory and inspiratory performance.
5. Give oxygen at 28%.
6. Limit activities until cardiovascular performance improves.
7. Monitor effects of diuretic; fluid intake and output; daily weights.

Cause 2
Chest infection. Propensity to bronchitis would make this likely, although sputum appears clear and frothy.

Expected outcome
Either eliminate chest infection as a cause or resolve with treatment within 5 days.

Interventions
1. Sputum cultures should be taken.
2. Physiotherapy and expectoration should be carried out.

Question 1

Now try to record on a separate sheet of paper at least two other possible causes of increasing breathlessness with their expected outcomes and interventions.

Problem 2

Increasing weakness; can only just move in bed but cannot get up and walk unaided.

Cause 1
Muscle tissue hypoxia related to impaired alveolar gas exchange and decreased tissue perfusion (result of decreased cardiac output).

Expected outcomes
Demonstrate a gradual ability to walk for further distances day by day, for example walk around the bed, walk to the lavatory.

Interventions
1. Controlled pattern of rest and activity, starting with more rest than activity. To have adequate rest after each activity.
2. Ensure that the patient is informed about the need for rest.

Cause 2
Inadequate diet; lack of calories and nutrients, particularly protein.

Expected outcome
Will be able to eat small nutritious meals within 1 week.

Interventions
1. Monitor food and fluid intake.
2. Initially give warm milk drinks or whatever she prefers. (Daily weights will be misleading as fluid is lost.)
3. Refer to dietician for a high-protein high-energy diet.
4. Give frequent small amounts of drink or food.

Cause 3
Electrolyte imbalance. Low potassium levels which may result from diuretic therapy cause weakness.

Expected outcome
Electrolyte levels within normal in 3 days.

Interventions
Supplements should be increased. Pineapple juice may be favoured by Mrs Jones. Low-sodium diet or fluids may be necessary when diet is resumed.

Question 2

Now try to record on a separate sheet of paper at least one other possible cause with expected outcomes and interventions.

Problem 3

Venous ulcer on right outer calf (size, 30 mm × 45 mm).

Cause
Increased venous and capillary pressure in lower leg, eventually resulting in impaired oxygen diffusion, and cellular and tissue breakdown (Browse, 1982).
   Oedema will exacerbate the problem.

Expected outcomes
1. Reduction in leg oedema as shown by weight reduction and calf measurements.
2. Reduction in ulcer size.
3. Presence of granulation tissue.

Interventions
1. Measure calves and weigh Mrs Jones daily.
2. Monitor diuretic therapy.
3. Keep legs elevated, but with caution as has heart failure.
4. Mobilise as soon as possible.
5. Granuflex dressing to be changed as frequently as indicated by discharge.
6. Compression bandage, or graduated Tubigrip.
7. Map ulcer on Cellophane paper every 3 days.

Question 3

Now on a separate sheet try to record at least one other possible cause of an ulcer.

Question 4

Try to identify, from the profile and assessment information, three further problems that might occur for this patient.

Rationale

Having identified the problems, the causes, the outcomes that we wish to achieve and the interventions that we need to make, let us now look at the rationale behind the care.

All treatments and activities should reflect the patient's own feelings and symptoms. With cardiac conditions in particular, a sensitive balance between rest and progressive activity should be determined by the patient's own energy levels (Shepherd, 1981). In an elderly patient such as Mrs Jones, skeletal muscle wasting will have advanced over several years as maximal activity levels may not have been at more than a basic level of independence. Lung function is also not likely to be very good owing to oedema and infections. Nursing care should therefore be gauged on the level of symptoms and by a realistic assessment of what might possibly be achieved to satisfy the patient's wishes.

Aims for the hospital stay should be as follows:

1. Reducing oxygen requirements of the body by:
   a. Rest
   b. Upright positioning.
   c. Oxygen therapy.

2. Maximising cardiac function by:
   a. Digitalis therapy.
   b. Diuretics.
   c. Balancing electrolytes.

Promoting rest for patients in hospital is a fundamental nursing function. Yet patients complain of noise, disturbance and inability to sleep (Wilson-Barnett, 1979). For patients like Mrs Jones, a rest schedule should be planned and, where possible, care, treatments, investigations and consultations should occur outside rest periods. Nighttime sleep is also essential, and alleviation of dyspnoea and discomfort may be enough to promote sleep. If this is not so, a light hypnotic such as temazepam may be offered. Mrs Jones will probably know all too well what helps her to rest and sleep and of course she should choose when she rests.

Limb weakness may not be helped by bed rest. Passive leg exercises and massage should be considered if bed rest continues for longer than a few days. As Fordham (1983) has discussed, it is a case of balancing all the body's needs for total rest without causing deconditioning of certain muscle groups. However, cardiac and lung function should be improved first before attending to skeletal muscles.

Oedema occurs when there is an excess of body water and sodium retained in the extra-cellular space. In normal tissues there is a negative extracellular fluid pressure and cells are held in close proximity to facilitate the exchange of gases, nutrients and waste products between cells and capillaries. If fluid accumulates, a positive extracellular pressure develops, prohibiting normal transfer be-tween cells. Hence, skin tissue cells can be dehydrated despite excess extracellular fluid and so Mrs Jones' skin appeared to be dry and inelastic. The diuretic therapy aims to remove excess fluid and sodium and to reduce extracellular pressure in order to promote correct hydration and nutrition of the tissues.

Mrs Jones' poor peripheral circulation, low arterial oxygen pressure and poor venous return have caused peripheral tissue break-down. Eliminating oedema, increasing oxygenation and facilitating venous return by leg elevation should promote healing. Sometimes, an infection may impede this.

A hydrocolloid dressing such as Granuflex has the properties that are considered de-sirable for wound dressings (Lawrence, 1985):

1. Protect wound from physical damage.
2. Exclude micro-organisms from the wound.
3. Prevent transfer of wound micro-organisms and exudate from the wound to the en-vironment.
4. To ensure patient comfort.

This type of dressing can be effective in reducing ulcer size and promoting healing (Ryan, 1985). It should be used according to the maker's instructions.

Tracing an ulcer can be an immensely im-portant activity. It prevents staff 'argument' about whether or not the ulcer is getting smaller, and obvious progress encourages the patient to keep the legs elevated. Tracing should not be done too often as a map with dated outlines is impossible to see clearly. Depending on the size of the ulcer and its healing rate, mapping once or twice a week may suffice.

Patients such as Mrs Jones learn to cope with disability in various ways. She has had medication for several years and is quite familiar with the main types and aims of treatment. Yet she may realise that her general deterioration is threatening her independence and domestic situation. The nurses must ensure Mrs Jones' sociability and easy manner does not mean they ignore her potential fundamental fears and worries. Full participation in discussions on care and plans for the future should be made possible if one or two nurses are made responsible for Mrs Jones' nursing care.

Evaluation

We have tackled three problems, based on the profile information, and con-sidered the rationale behind that care. How effective has it been? In this section, we evaluate that care.

Problem 1

Increasing breathlessness.
Causes 1 appeared the most relevant. No chest infection was isolated.

3 days after admission:
1. The respiration rate is 25/min, without any additional oxygen.
2. Mrs Jones can talk more easily and seems more comfortable.
3. The pulse is still somewhat irregular but seems stronger (digoxin was increased to 125 μg a day); the blood pressure is 120/70 mmHg.

7 days after admission:
1. The respiration rate is 18/min.

2. Mrs Jones can walk slowly up the ward.
3. The pulse is usually regular at 70.

Problem 2

Increasing weakness.
First week after admission:

1. Mrs Jones can manage to walk up the ward but has to rest before washing or using the lavatory.
2. Mrs Jones feels that she probably could manage to make a cup of tea if she were at home, although the nurses feel that this would be quite a strain.
3. Mrs Jones appreciates her hour's rest before lunch and mid-afternoon.
4. She has become much more independent in washing.

Problem 3

Leg ulcer.
Swabs reveal no infection or abnormal cells.
4 days after admission:

1. Calf size is decreasing after 4 days. The calves appear less oedematous.
2. Ulcer mapping is successfully demonstrating a reduction in ulcer size, which is very encouraging for Mrs Jones and the nurses.
3. Her weight is now 52 kg.
4. The ulcer is clean and granulating.
5. Mrs Jones tolerates the treatment well.

7 days after admission:

1. No change in calf size.
2. Dimensions of ulcer reduced.
3. Weight is 50 kg.

Answers to questions 1, 2, 3 and 4

Problem 1

Question 1

Other causes of increasing breathlessness might include the following.

Cause 1
Anxiety; possibly Mrs Jones was worried about leaving her home, about the new treatments and new staff.

Expected outcome
That, by day 2, Mrs Jones will not look anxious and that her breathlessness will resolve.

Intervention
Careful discussions, and one nurse (her primary nurse) will try to get to know Mrs Jones well and to understand any worries. Sensitive information-giving and introductions to other patients may help.

Cause 2
Atrial fibrillation.

Expected outcome
Deficit reduced by 5/min.

Intervention
Increased digoxin dose, which should reduce deficit.

93

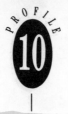
Problem 2

Question 2

Other causes of increasing weakness might include the following.

Cause

Heaviness of limbs. It appears so much more difficult for Mrs Jones to move her legs as they are so heavy owing to fluid retention.

Expected outcome

That, by day 3, the oedema will have re-solved; calf girth will have reduced by 1 in each day and that Mrs Jones' weight will be down to 52 kg.

Intervention

Support limbs; administer diuretics; weigh daily.

Problem 3

Question 3

One other possible cause of leg ulcers is a malignant growth. In Mrs Jones' case, it is unlikely that her ulcer is malignant because of her previous ulcer history.

The three further problems are as follows.

Problem 4

Question 4

Immobility.

Cause

Lack of strength of patient.

Expected outcome

Patient will become more mobile, as planned for Problem 2.

Intervention

To prevent pressure sores, patient to rest in bed on a sheepskin. Physiotherapy to be given to help to prevent chest infection and deep vein thrombosis.

PROFILE 10

Problem 5

Constipation.

Cause
Inadequate diet.

Expected outcome
That Mrs Jones' bowels will open regularly
every other day as is 'normal' for her.

Intervention
A controlled diet, with adequate roughage.
4 days after admission her bowels opened
once and patient felt comfortable but suppositories had to be given. By 7 days, her
bowels had opened three times.

Problem 6

Being able to cope at home.

Cause
Difficulty in getting round the house,
weakness and breathlessness.

Expected outcome
That Mrs Jones will be ready and prepared
to be discharged within 2 weeks of her
admission.

Intervention
Care must be aimed towards enabling Mrs
Jones to have maximum independence.
The social worker to visit, and the district
nurse to be contacted to talk to Mrs Jones
and her primary nurse. Primary nurse is
also to talk to Mrs Jones' friend 'across the
way'.

References

Browse, N. L., and Burnard, K. G. (1982). The cause of venous
ulceration. *The Lancet*, **2**, 243–245.
Fordham, M. (1983). In: Wilson-Barnett, J., and Fordham, M.
(eds), *Recovery from Illness*, Wiley, Chichester, West Sussex,
Chapter 1.
Lawrence, J. C. (1985). The physical properties of a new hydro-
colloid dressing. In: Ryan, T. J. (ed.), *Royal Society of Medicine
International Congress and Symposium Series*, Royal Society of

Medicine, London.
Ryan, T. J. (ed.) (1985). An environment for healing: the role of
occlusion. *Royal Society of Medicine International Congress and
Symposium Series*, Royal Society of Medicine, London.
Shepherd, R. J. (1981). *Ischaemic Heart Disease and Exercise*,
Croom Helm, London.
Wilson-Barnett, J. (1979). *Stress in Hospital*, Churchill Living-
stone, Edinburgh.

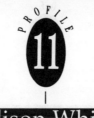

Alison While

A handicapped child admitted to hospital to improve her mobility skills:

Planning care to improve walking and other self-care activities

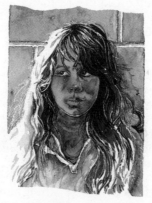

12-*year-old Sarah has spastic quadriplegia and has been admitted to hospital to improve her mobility skills. She is also handicapped mentally. Some of the problems associated with Sarah's condition are outlined and the way in which the nursing team will intervene to ensure that Sarah will be able to fulfil her maximum potential is given. Further problems need to be identified, together with the interventions necessary; the answers are at the end of the chapter.*

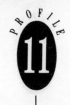

Patient profile

Sarah Jackson is 12 years old and was admitted to hospital to improve her mobility skills. She has mobility problems because of her spastic quadriplegia and her difficulties are increased by moderate mental handicap (IQ, 20–50 range). Sarah was admitted from the waiting list, as out-patient supervision and physiotherapy at school had failed to yield significant improvements in her mobility skills. Lack of safe mobility has been identified as inhibiting the development of Sarah's independence in daily living activities.

Assessment information
Biographical and social information
Sarah is the youngest of two daughters by several years. Her parents were divorced in October 1985 and her mother, with whom she lives during the school holidays, is a housewife. The family live in a two-bedroom council flat about 6 miles from the hospital.

Sarah has been classified as educationally subnormal (severe) since an early age. At the age of 3 months, she suffered severe epileptic fits which were later diagnosed as infantile spasms and were said to have caused cerebral atrophy. She has been attending a special boarding school in southern England for the past 4 years.

Sarah has no contact with her father.

Current health status
Sarah falls frequently, even when walking with a rollator. Before orthopaedic surgery, she had fixed flexion at her knees and limited extension of the hips and everted feet. According to Sarah, she has come into hospital to learn how to stand and walk properly. Her mother has a similar understanding of the aims of hospital admission. Sarah has no other health problems.

Assessment
Safety in the environment
Sarah's safety is clearly an important consideration. She attends a special school where there is full supervision of her activities. However, her walking difficulties result in her falling frequently. She has a limited appreciation of dangers in her environment. Her mother provides full-time care during the holidays.

Communicating
Sarah's communication skills reflect her limited intellectual ability. She has a small vocabulary and her poor pronunciation makes it difficult to understand what she is saying and the depth of her understanding. Throughout conversation, Sarah refers to her 'baby', a soft doll called Tom. It is therefore difficult to gain Sarah's co-operation in her care and, since her mother visits her only during the evening, she cannot offer more than transient help.

Emotional state
Sarah states that she would rather be at school with her friends. She says that the only person who really cares for her is her doll Tom. She appears bored and rather lonely and looks forward to seeing her mother every evening.

Eating and drinking
Sarah weighs 40.3 kg and is 1.46 m tall. She enjoys her meal times and claims to like anything although she has difficulty eating some foods without help because her manual dexterity is poor. Her favourite drink is Ribena and, like all children, she is fond of sweets.

Eliminating
Sarah is dependent upon others for personal cleansing although she is able to assist with her daily bath. She enjoys having her hair washed and likes her long brown hair brushed and plaited. She can dress herself with assistance; she cannot manage buttons or shoe laces. Unless reminded and supervised, Sarah would neglect to clean her teeth.

Mobilising
Orthopaedic surgery has improved the position of her knees and hips but her

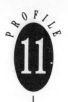
muscular development and control are very poor. Her spasticity gives her a staggering gait and she needs to learn how she may best achieve safe ambulation within her limited potential. She is unable to stand without assistance and cannot maintain an upright position without physical support. Sarah takes large slithering strides, rarely lifting her feet properly and easily becoming unbalanced. She cannot accomplish turning or transfer to a chair safely.

Working and playing
As already stated, Sarah attends a special boarding school, returning to her mother's care during the school holidays. She has a limited span of concentration—a maximum of 10 min on a short task. Sarah seems to enjoy her schooling. She states that her favourite games include playing with her doll Tom, blowing bubbles, doing jigsaws, painting and Plasticene modelling. She does not like books and states that she is bored in hospital.

Sleeping
Sarah sleeps soundly from 9.00 pm and wakes at about 6.00 am.

Problems, expected outcomes, and interventions

Problem 1

Frequent falls arising from Sarah's handicapped condition.

Causes
The position of Sarah's knees, hips and feet do not enable safe ambulation. Further, poor muscular development exacerbates her difficulties as does the spasticity of the muscles which limits her control over her leg movements. Sarah's limited intellectual ability has inhibited learning of necessary skills and her brain function is slow so that normal responses to the body's servo-mechanism are not operant.

Expected outcome
That Sarah will be able to stand safely and to walk slowly using a rollator.

Interventions
A team approach will be adopted, with the nurses reinforcing the exercises that Sarah has been taught by the physiotherapist.

The programme will include:
1. Good sleeping position at night.
2. Good resting positions during the day.
3. Wearing of suitable clothes and specially fitted support footwear.
4. Operant conditioning regarding the approach to walking, that is reward giving for careful attempts at standing and walking.
5. Instruction and practice will be given in:
   a. Rising from sitting to standing.
   b. Standing to sitting.
   c. Gaining good standing posture.
   d. Walking with a rollator.
6. For further information on walking retraining, see Chapter 5.

Question 1

On a separate sheet of paper, outline positions which would prevent deformity and allow cerebral palsied children to use and develop whatever movement abilities they have.

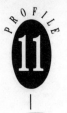
Problem 2

Separation anxiety arising from hospitalisation.

Causes

Sarah is in an unfamiliar environment; she is separated from her school-friends and her normal life routines and is unfamiliar with the hospital staff and the routines of hospital life. Her limited communication skills are increasing her feelings of isolation and make it more difficult for her to make sense of her environment.

Expected outcome

That Sarah will feel less lonely and identify with her 'special' nurse.

Interventions

1. A primary nurse will undertake Sarah's care as often as she is on duty.

2. An identified nurse will be allocated to look after Sarah during each shift. She should introduce herself and make sure that Sarah knows how to attract her attention.
3. Sarah's allocated nurse will set aside at least 1 hour of each nursing shift to play with Sarah.
4. Sarah's visitors will be warmly welcomed to the ward and her mother invited to participate in Sarah's care as much as possible.

Question 2

On a separate sheet of paper, list any other interventions which would ameliorate separation anxiety.

Problem 3

Interruption of educational programme owing to hospitalisation.

Cause

A paediatric ward in a general hospital is unaccustomed to furthering the skill acquisition of mentally handicapped children.

Expected outcome

That Sarah will show continued gain in social and cognitive behaviours.

Interventions

The educational programme will include:

1. Organised opportunities for Sarah to talk with others. Nurses will reinforce and encourage attempts to extend her vocabulary.

2. Assessment of incontinence pattern and development of lavatory routine to create a habitual routine for defaecation and micturition. Sarah will be rewarded for performing successfully.
3. Organised opportunities for Sarah to develop further her skills of independent living. Nurses will encourage Sarah to wash her hands, the front of her trunk and her face during bathing, to brush her teeth after breakfast and after her last meal of the day, to brush her hair, to dress and undress herself and to feed herself with as little mess as possible. She will be rewarded for performing successfully.

Question 3

Design a detailed programme to teach a mentally handicapped child handwashing.

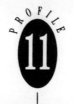
Rationale

Physical handicap is not infrequently associated with moderate and severe mental handicap and, where these handicaps occur together, the individual needs much good care so that she may fulfil her maximum potential (Committee on Mental Handicap Nursing and Care, 1979). Unlike normal children, those who are cerebral palsied need assistance in adopting body positioning which will prevent the development of deformity (Nicoll, 1984). However, much research has demonstrated that community support for families with handicapped children is limited (Hewett *et al.*, 1970; Wilkin, 1979; Tarran, 1981) and many cerebral palsied children consequently develop deformity which requires correction in later life if they are to develop their skills in independent living.

Sarah has already had orthopaedic correction of her acquired hip and leg deformities; so it is imperative that she is taught exercises to develop her leg muscle control and to gain safe mobility skills. Correct positioning of the body at rest has been demonstrated to prevent deformities (Nicoll, 1984) and a child with moderate mental handicap may be assisted in adopting good positions. Unlike normal individuals, those with a cerebral palsy do not have the same control over voluntary muscles and have to be taught how to stand and walk, using an aid appropriately where necessary. While children with normal intellect may receive reward from achievement of a task, operant conditioning is frequently used in the field of mental handicap to encourage the acquisition of skills (Blackman, 1974).

Separation anxiety is commonly experienced by children admitted to hospital and tends to be more severe among younger and more dependent children, especially where parental contact is limited (MacCarthy, 1981). The detrimental effects of separation from the family was the concern of the Platt Report (Ministry of Health, Central Health Services Council, 1959) which, among its many recommendations, suggested that hospital care should acknowledge the very particular needs of children. Hawthorn's (1974) study revealed that children in hospital spend much of their time on their own and that they are frequently miserable. Jolly (1981) has many helpful suggestions to improve nursing care, and she and others stress the importance of explaining all procedures carefully to children (Rodin, 1983). The limited understanding that children have of hospital life has been described by Eiser and Patterson (1984) and the use of play to reduce anxiety is important (Petrillo and Sanger, 1980).

Mentally handicapped individuals have an impaired ability to acquire new knowledge and skills (Clarke and Clarke, 1974) and therefore no opportunity should be lost in promoting learning. There is evidence that institutional care encourages the development of learned helplessness (Tierney, 1983); so every care must be taken to ensure that learning continues. Social skills, to a large extent, are dependent upon the acquisition of good communication skills, and mentally handicapped people frequently need additional help in acquiring them (Clarke and Clarke, 1974).

Incontinence causes additional strains on family life and, where continence is achieved, a child's overall management is much easier and more easily sustained in the community.

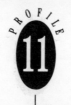
Evaluation

Problem 1

Frequent falls.

Acquisition of safe walking skills will occur over an extended period. However, Sarah's progress should be evaluated at weekly intervals and Sarah reminded of her progress. The following criteria may be used:

1. The body position adopted by Sarah when sleeping at night; in particular, whether she is beginning to adopt a more extended body position.
2. The care taken by Sarah in gaining a standing position and the success that she has in gaining a good standing position without falling.
3. Later, the evaluation should include acquisition of safe walking skills.

Problem 2

Separation anxiety.

Sarah's emotional state should be evaluated every 2–3 days so that her hospital stay involves as little unhappiness as possible and she is able to gain from her experience.

The following criteria may be used:

1. Sarah's statements regarding her state of well-being, for example whether she is lonely and whether she feels that only her doll Tom cares for her.
2. Sarah's general confidence in dealing with the nursing staff and whether she identifies with a particular nurse and derives pleasure from the relationship.
3. Sarah's willingness to co-operate with nursing and other staff.

Problem 3

Interruption of education.

Sarah's progress should not have been interrupted by her hospitalisation. Her continued progress in the acquisition of skills of independent living should be evaluated weekly and the educational programme adapted to reflect her progress and to continue her skill acquisition.

The following criteria may be used:

1. Sarah's verbal articulation and appropriateness; acquisition of new words and their appropriate use.
2. Sarah's ability at self-care, for example handwashing, teeth brushing, hair care, dressing and undressing, and tidy feeding.

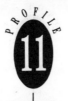

Answers to questions 1, 2 and 3

Problem 1

Question 1

Positions which would prevent deformity are:

1. The prone position. This prevents the development of a curled-up position and can be used to practise lifting of the head and taking weight on elbows and hands. This position allows the person to use his hands together and to co-ordinate hand and eye.

2. The side position is useful because it helps to prevent the cerebral palsied person from arching his back and becoming stiff.

3. A well-supported sitting position promotes trunk and pelvic stability which is important if head control is to be gained. It also frees the hands for use. Correct support is important so that the legs and hips do not fall to one side.

Problem 2

Question 2

Other interventions to reduce separation anxiety might include:

1. Use of familiar words for everyday activities; special words for use of lavatory, for example.
2. Adherence to home routines as much as possible.

3. All procedures involving the child should be carefully explained using appropriate language, line drawings, books and toys. A familiar person should be present during stressful procedures.
4. All visitors should be welcomed to the ward and invited to visit frequently.
5. Play sessions; these allow children to express their anxieties and work through their feelings.

Problem 3

Question 3

The programme for teaching a mentally handicapped child handwashing should include teaching the child:

1. To place the plug in the basin.

2. To be able to control the water tap.
3. To be able to pick up the soap.
4. To be able to lather and rinse her hands.
5. To be able to find the towel and to dry her hands.
6. To leave the basin clean.

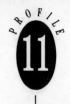

References

Blackman, D. (1974). *Operant Conditioning*, Methuen, London.

Clarke, A. M., and Clarke, A. D. B. (eds) (1974). *Readings from Mental Deficiency: The Changing Outlook*, Methuen, London.

Committee on Mental Handicap Nursing and Care (1979). *Report of the Committee on Mental Handicap Nursing and Care* (Jay Report), Cmnd 7468, HMSO, London.

Eiser, C., and Patterson, D. (1984). Children's perceptions of hospital: a preliminary study. *International Journal of Nursing Studies*, **21**, 45–50.

Hawthorn, P. J. (1974). *Nurse—I want My Mummy!*, Royal College of Nursing, London.

Hewett, S., Newson, J., and Newson, E. (1970). *The Family and the Handicapped Child*, Allen and Unwin, London.

Jolly, J. (1981). *The Other Side of Paediatrics*, Macmillan, London.

MacCarthy, D. (1981). The under-fives in hospital. *Nursing Times*, **77** (30), suppl., 1–8.

Ministry of Health, Central Health Services Council (1959). *The Welfare of Children in Hospital*, (Platt Report) HMSO, London.

Nicoll, A. (1984). Preventing deformity in severe cerebral palsy I and II. *Maternal and Child Health*, **9** (6), 191–193; **9** (7), 224–227.

Petrillo, M., and Sanger, S. (1980). *Emotional Care of Hospitalised Children*, Lippincott, Philadelphia, Pennsylvania.

Rodin, J. (1983). *Will This Hurt?*, Royal College of Nursing, London.

Tarran, E. C. (1981). Parents' views of medical and social work services for families with a young cerebral-palsied child. *Developmental Medicine and Child Neurology*, **23**, 173–182.

Tierney, A. J. (ed.) (1983). *Nurses and the Mentally Handicapped*, John Wiley, Chichester, West Sussex.

Wilkin, D. (1979). *Caring for the Mentally Handicapped Child*, Croom Helm, London.

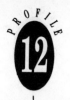

Lynn Batehup and Jenifer Wilson-Barnett

Conclusion

In reviewing these 11 chapters, which are aimed at exploring problem identification and planning interventions, several aspects of the nursing process and knowledge base become clear. It is obvious for example that a wide range of problems can be identified for this small group of individuals. They span the entire range of biological responses which have implications for nursing care. Some are more clearly delineated and have only one cause and consequence, such as the venous stasis ulcer, while others may be caused by many causal agents and result in a complex picture of disability, such as anxiety or difficulty in coping with others after taking an overdose.

It is extremely difficult to categorise problems and interventions discussed in these chapters because several problems span more than one category, such as sleep problems and poor appetite. However, an attempt will be made in order to emphasise certain features for which we are responsible. Other issues, such as the role of nursing interventions in the overall plan of work by the team, also tend to raise questions about how much we can initiate our own treatments or replicate other specialists' therapies.

Problems fall into six major categories, but the reader must always acknowledge that these are not discrete categories. As we know, physical problems may have several implications for and influence psychological responses, while enduring psychological problems can ultimately cause physical and social difficulties.

The physical problems in Table 12.1 are basic; they are physical problems that had serious and distressing consequences for the individuals concerned. All required detailed assessments to identify causal factors and to plan care, but the interventions recommended for the majority involved quite practical strategies. Changes in posture and in positioning of furniture as well as continuous explanation, monitoring and

Table 12.1 Physical problems

Problem	Chapter
Propensity to fall	5
Incontinence	5
Difficulty in walking	11
Breathlessness	10
Weakness	10
Venous stasis ulcer	10

Table 12.2 Problems with comfort

Problem	Chapter
Sleep deprivation	4
Poor appetite and nausea	6
Pain	4, 6

Table 12.3 Potential physical problems due to long-term illness

Problem	Chapter
Possible permanent deformity through immobility	8
Possible respiratory depression	7
Possible infection through reduced resistance	6
At risk of pressure sores due to immobility	9

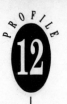

schedules for exercise and rest were needed. After other staff were also initially involved in recommending strategies, nurses and their clients were the ones who were accountable for putting these into action.

'Comfort care' (Table 12.2) is one of the most vital areas of nursing and tends to be used as an adjunct to other more conventional means of alleviating pain or discomfort. As well as using standard measures, such as pharmacological agents, narcotics, anti-emetics and analgesics, nurses really need to study other alternatives.

Part of the nurses' role is preventative (Table 12.3), that is identifying potential problems and reducing the risk of these by planning and providing appropriate care. So many of the chronic illnesses that befall our patient population could be prevented by reducing risk factors earlier in life but, while we need to spend more time in promoting health for younger people, secondary-problem prevention for those in older age already occupies a great deal of nursing time. From these chapters, it seems that monitoring the risk status and levels of certain substances is a vital responsibility for both nurses and doctors. However, positioning and reposi-tioning those who are partially mobile is essential nursing to prevent malalignment of limbs, after a stroke and pressure sores, both of which can delay or impede recovery com-pletely.

So often now, chronic degenerative dis-orders are treated with surgery, and there-fore post-operative nursing must take account of increased likelihood of post-operative complications (Table 12.4). Cardiac and thoracic surgery are typical examples of major interventions with great potential benefit to patients. However, poor circulation is already established for the first case, which may make healing difficult and the removal of an infected lobe obviously puts healthy tissue at risk of contamination. Clean environments, adequate hydration and diet, wound care and exercises are all prescribed, but nurses need vigilance in helping both patients and relatives to be actively involved and in-formed of these essential components in care.

Psychological care (Table 12.5) is needed for all those with health problems, be they explicitly psychological, that is a disturbance in thought or emotion, or physical. Benefits which have been documented include an improved mental and physical status. How-ever, the wide range of problems identified across the 11 chapters indicate that psycho-logical factors are relevant to most subjects; the six identified are therefore a conservative assessment. This demonstrates how impor-tant psychological care is, both in preventing such problems and in helping subjects to cope when they occur.

Table 12.4 Potential physical problems after surgery

Problem	Chapter
Wound infection	4, 9
Lung collapse from bleeding in the pleural cavity	9
Chest infection	4, 9

Table 12.5 Psychosocial problems

Problem	Chapter
Separation anxiety	7, 11
Anxiety over effects of illness	1, 4
Unwilling to communicate	7
Concern about the reactions of others to one's 'irresponsible' behaviour	7
Disturbed self-concept after major surgery	9
Post-natal depression	3

Table 12.6 Problems due to poor understanding and adjustment

Problem	Chapter
Addiction to smoking	1
Unsocial behaviour	11
Poor management of diabetes	2
Difficulties with breastfeeding	3

Psychosocial interventions are often not explained very fully, as it is somewhat difficult to operationalise such interventions. What does seem crucial to the needs of all these subjects is time with a nurse who gives an adequate opportunity to listen and thereby to show care for her troubled patient. In the general ward, so much psychological morbidity goes unrecognised that it is essential to include problems on the care plan and purposefully to provide time to give this care. Listening, supporting and explaining tend to form the basis of usual nursing psychological care. Communication skills and warmth are essential to incorporate these aspects naturally within the role of a nurse.

For some, deep emotional problems may require referral to a psychiatrist, but an essential adjunct to this can be provided by a nurse or close relative who provides the continuous presence of someone who shows they care. Perhaps one of our major challenges in the general care setting is to provide time for this, reflecting the high priority that it should receive. Few others are so well placed or prepared to cope with such problems in the hospital setting.

Problems related to poor understanding and adjustment (Table 12.6) require an educational approach by the nurse, that is not only in giving information relevant to the problem, but also in discussing with subjects their own perception of the problem and their own understanding and wishes. There is no doubt that, as health care professionals, we have not been very adept at 'teaching' in the past, using rather out-dated modes of information presentation and hoping for out-

comes akin to 'compliance'. More sympathetic and realistic approaches have been demonstrably more effective in helping subjects to identify their own wishes and plans for changing their behaviour. Participation in treatment and discussion is called for; where possible, it tends to help clients to understand their responsibilities and all the team to agree on more realistic targets.

Operant conditioning may be appropriate for those with learning problems or addictions and should be used sensitively when appropriate. Other educational interventions tend to be enhanced when relatives and sometimes groups with similar needs are included. Nurses then learn to become facilitators and participants rather than teachers. Previously recovered patients are often invaluable as supporters for those who are struggling to adapt.

In all these 11 chapters, real 'clients' or 'patients' have been described so that their problems are not artificial. Clearly, some are more easily 'assessed' and 'processed' than others, most patients tending to have several problems for which there may be several interventions. Rationales for care demonstrate that much more research is needed to guide practice. Hopefully, others will be familiar with useful studies and thereby will improve interventions and methods for evaluation. Just as many clients may be helped by participating in treatment, decisions and plans, we hope that readers of this book will be active, not only in completing the gaps and answers, but also in asking new questions and using this approach when analysing the care that they give their patients.

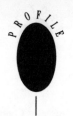

Subject Index

Accommodation, unsuitable, problem of, 61, 62
N-Acetylcysteine, 59
Alcohol, as cause of respiratory depression, 56, 59–60, 61, 64
Alcoholic liver disease, 11–12
Angina, unstable, 27–34
Anxiety
  over effects of illness, 3ff, 33, 52
  separation, 57, 61, 62, 100ff
  about social service involvement, 62
Appetite, poor, 47–8, 49, 50
Assessment, general comments on, ix–x, xiii
  of activity after stroke, 68, 73
  of micturition pattern, 42
  of pain, 30, 49, 51
  of pressure-sore risk, 85
Association of Breastfeeding Mothers, 25
Atenolol, 2

Balance mechanism, 38, 39
  impairment of, 40
  retraining after stroke, 73
Beclamethasone inhaler, 80
Bleeding in pleural cavity, lung collapse from, potential, 81–3
Blood glucose levels, see Diabetes management
BM Stix, 13, 64
Bone metastases after mastectomy, 45–52
Breast cancer, symptom control in, 45–52
Breastfeeding, difficulties with, 19–26
Breathlessness, 28, 89, 92–3
Bronchiectasis, 83

Cancer, see Breast cancer, symptom control, in
Cardiac surgery to relieve unstable angina, 27–34
Cerebral palsy, see Mobility skills of handicapped child, improvement of
Charcoal, 59
Chemotherapy, cytotoxic, side-effects of, 45ff
Chest infection after surgery, potential, 82, 84
Comfort, problems with, 105, 106
  pain, 30ff, 48ff
  poor appetite and nausea, 47ff

sleep deprivation, 29, 31, 32
Communication problems, 55, 60, 100, 101
Constipation, 95
Control over life-style and body function, perceived loss of, 52
Coronary artery bypass graft, see Coronary vein graft surgery
Coronary vein graft surgery, 27–34
Counselling after myocardial infarction, 3ff
CRYSIS, 25
Cytotoxic chemotherapy, side-effects of, 45ff

Deep vein thrombosis after stroke, 71–2
Deformity, permanent, possible, due to immobility, 69ff
Depression after stroke, 72, 76
Diabetes management, 9–17
Diet modification, 5
Dietary control in diabetes, 13
Digoxin, 88, 92, 93
Domperidone, 50
Drug overdose, 53–65

Educational programme of handicapped child, interruption of, owing to hospitalisation, 100, 102
Emotionalism after stroke, 72, 76
Evaluation, general comments on, xii-xiii
Exercise, lack of, 6
'Expected outcome', definition of, xi

Falls, frequent, 35–43, 99, 101, 102
Flaccidity after stroke, 69, 71
Frusemide, 88

Glucose, blood, see Diabetes management
Glyceryl trinitrate, 28
Granuflex, 92

Health education after myocardial infarction, 3ff
Heart attack, see Myocardial infarction, rehabilitation after

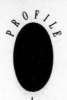

Heart failure, successful recovery from, planning for, 87–95
Helplessness, feelings of, 57, 61, 62, 64
Hepatotoxicity, 56, 59, 60, 63
Hypercalcaemia, 47, 48, 49
Hyperglycaemia, 14, 15
Hypoglycaemia, 13–14, 15, 59, 60

Immobility
    following heart failure, 94
    as possible cause of permanent deformity, 69ff
    as possible cause of pressure sores, 85–6
Incontinence, 37ff, 101
Indomethacin, 47, 50
Infection, possible
    of chest, 82
    through reduced resistance, 51
    of umbilical cord, 22ff
    of wound, 30 ff, 84–5
Insulin, 10ff
Intermediate-acting insulin, 10
Interventions, general comments on, xii
Isosorbide dinitrate, 28

Ketodiastix, 10

Lactation, adequate, establishment of, 21ff
Leg ulcer, 90, 92, 93, 94
Leukopenia, 51
Life-style and body function, control over, perceived loss of, 52
Liver disease, alcoholic, 11–12
Lobectomy, acute post-operative period of, planning in, 79–86
Lung collapse, potential, 81, 82, 84

Malalignment of shoulder after stroke, 69, 71
Mastectomy, bone metastases after, 45 ff
Mental handicap, see Mobility skills of handicapped child, improvement of
Methionine, 56, 59
Mixtard insulin, 10
Mobility
    impaired, after stroke, 70
    safe, planning for, 35–43
Mobility assessment after stroke, 68, 74
Mobility skills of handicapped child, improvement of, 97–104
Morphine sulphate, 47, 50, 51
Myocardial infarction, rehabilitation after, 1–7

Nausea, 47–8, 49, 50

Oedema, 90, 92, 93, 94
Outcomes, general comments on, xi–xii

Overdose patients, see Drug overdose
Oxytocin, 23

Pain, 30, 31, 32, 48, 49, 50, 51
Pancreatic insufficiency, 11–12
Paracetamol overdose, 53–65
Parasuicides, see Drug overdose
Parvolex, 59
Physical problems, 105–6
    breathlessness, 89, 92–3
    incontinence, 37ff, 101
    potential, due to long-term illness
        possible hepatic impairment through toxicity, 56, 59, 60, 63
        possible infection through reduced resistance, 51
        possible permanent deformity through immobility, 69ff
        possible respiratory depression, 56, 61, 63–4
        risk of pressure sores due to immobility, 85–6
    potential, after surgery, 106
        chest infection, 82, 84
        lung collapse, 81, 82, 84
        wound infection, 30ff, 82, 84–5
    potential infection of umbilical cord, 22ff
    propensity to fall, 35–43, 99, 101, 102
    venous ulcer, 90ff
    walking difficulties, 97–104 (see also under Mobility)
    weakness, 90, 91, 93, 94
    weight difficulties, 4ff
Physical stress, role of, in raising blood sugar levels, 13, 15–16
Poor understanding and adjustment, problems due to, 107
    addiction to smoking, 3ff
    difficulties with breastfeeding, 21ff
    poor management of diabetes, 9ff
    unsocial behaviour, 101
'Post-fall syndrome', 40, 42
Post-natal depression, 22, 23–4, 25
Post-operative wound infection, potential, 30ff, 84–5
Postural balance mechanism, impairment of, after stroke, 70
Postural control, loss of, 38ff
Potassium, slow release, 88
Pressure sores due to immobility, risk of, 85–6
Problems, specific, see Comfort, problems with; Physical problems; Poor understanding and adjustment, problems due to; Psychosocial problems
Problem statements, general comments on, x–xi
Prolactin, 23
Psychological stress, role of, in raising blood sugar levels, 13, 15–16

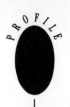

Psychosocial problems, 106–7
  anxiety over effects of illness, 3ff, 52
  concern about reactions of others to one's irres-
    ponsible behaviour, 59–60
  disturbed self-concept after major surgery, 85
  post-natal depression, 22, 23–4, 25
  separation anxiety, 57, 61, 62, 100ff
  unwillingness to communicate, 55, 60

Radiotherapy, side-effects of, 49
Rehabilitation
  in acute stage of recovery from stroke, 67–77
  after coronary vein graft surgery, 31, 33
  after myocardial infarction, 1–7
Resistance, reduced, possible infection through,
  51
Respiratory depression, possible, 56, 61, 63–4
Rumack-Matthews nomogram for paracetamol
  poisoning, 59

Safe mobility, planning for, 35–43
Salbutamol inhaler, 80
Self-concept, disturbance of, after lobectomy, 85
Separation anxiety, 57, 61, 62, 100ff
Servomechanism, body's, for prevention of falls,
  38, 39–40
Shoulder malalignment and subluxation after
  stroke, 69, 71
Sleep deprivation, 29, 31, 32
Slow release potassium, 88
Smoking, addiction to, 3ff
Social service involvement, anxiety about, 62
Spasticity after stroke, 69, 71
Spastic quadriplegia, see Mobility skills of handi-
  capped child, improvement of

Sternotomy, see Cardiac surgery to relieve unstable
  angina
Stomach wash-out, 59–60, 63, 64
Stress, role of, in raising blood sugar levels, 13,
  15–16
Stroke, recovery from, acute stage of, rehabilitation
  in, 67–77
Subluxation of shoulder after stroke, 71
Surgery, major, disturbed self-concept after, 85
Surgery, potential physical problems after, 106
  chest infection, 82, 84
  lung collapse, 81, 82, 84
  wound infection, 30ff, 84–5

Toxicity, possible hepatic impairment through,
  56, 59, 60, 63

Ulcer, venous, 90, 92, 93, 94
Umbilical cord, infection of, potential, 22ff
Understanding and adjustment, poor, see Poor
  understanding and adjustment, problems due
  to
Unsocial behaviour, 101
Unstable angina, 27–34

Vein graft surgery, see Coronary vein graft surgery
Venous ulcer, 90, 92, 93, 94

Walking difficulties, 35ff, 97ff (see also under
  Mobility)
Walking retraining, post-fall, 41–2
Walking skills of handicapped child, improve-
  ment of, 97–104
Weakness, 90, 91, 93, 94
Weight difficulties, 4ff
Wound infection after surgery, potential, 30ff, 84–5